The
Enzyme Diet™
Solution

Finally, Weight Loss That Stays Lost™

Other books by Dr. Allan Somersall:

Your Very Good Health: 101 Healthy Lifestyle Choices

A Passion For Living: The Art of Real Success

Your Evolution to YES!

Understanding The Evolution of YES!

Evolutionary Tales by Dr. YES!

Breakthrough In Cell Defense

Nature's Goldmine

The
Enzyme Diet™
Solution

Finally, Weight Loss That Stays Lost™

How to use the **Power of Enzymes**
to obtain the Healthier Body you desire!

Allan C. Somersall, Ph.D., M.D.
with Jennifer B. Ferniza, M.S., CCN

The Natural Wellness Group
2-3415 Dixie Road, Suite: 538
Mississauga, Ontario L4Y 2B1
www.thenaturalwellnessgroup.com
1-800-501-8516
enzymedietbook@aol.com

The Natural Wellness Group is an Imprint of GOLDENeight Publishers

Library of Congress Cataloging-in-Publication Data # 2003101197

Available at Library of Congress

Includes Index.
ISBN #1-890412-98-8

Printed and bound in Canada

10   9   8   7   6   5   4   3   2

Somersall, Allan (Dr.)
    How to use the Power of Enzymes to obtain the Healthier Body you desire!
1. Diet   2. Weight loss   3. Health   4. Fitness

Cover design by Piper Group Inc.,
Edited by:
    Tania Sarrentino, M.S., CCN
    Ann-Marie Junor, B.Sc., B.Ed.
    Joy Kies

Enzyme Flavors courtesy of Susan B. Tucker

The Enzyme Diet™; *Finally, Weight Loss That Stays Lost*™ and CAeDS®are trademarks of Infinity2 Inc., Scottsdale, Arizona

❧   Dedicated to a trio of scientific pioneers   ❧

Dr. Stan Bynum

Dr. Edward Howell

Dr. Harvey Ashmead

℘   **Acknowledgements**   ℘

The principal author is indebted to a number of people who made many invaludable contributions to this book:

To Jennifer Ferniza who contributed significantly to the text, especially in Chapters 6, 7, 8 and 9. Her expertise and critical comments made the complete book what it is. For this contribution, she is duly recognized as a co-author;

To Drs. Stan Bynum, Edward Howell and Harvey Ashmead - three pioneer researchers who made The Enzyme Diet™ possible and to whom this book is dedicated;

To Paul Janson, Ann-Marie Junor, Tanya Sarrentino, Joy Kies and my wife, Virginia, for their valuable editing and comments;

To the creative designers at Piper Group for a most attractive cover design;

To Edward Hoyt for his support of this project;

To my dear family, for their patience, support and encouragement; and finally but most importantly,

To my agent, Carolina Loren for once again surpassing all my expectations by championing this new book, executing all the details of its evolution with finesse and guiding it through to completion.

To all of you, I am most grateful, for without such a favorable support cast, this book would not become a reality. In the final analysis, however, all the short-comings are mine. I thank you all most sincerely.

Dr. A.C. Somersall

Contents

PART III

YOUR PERSONAL APPLICATION
Are You Framing A Winning Plan?

DISCLAIMER

This book is designed to provide information to the public at large. Nothing herein is intended to advise or encourage the reader to practice any form of clinical self-diagnosis or treatment. Medical problems should always be addresseed by competent healthcare professionals on an individual basis. Pateints with obesity must therefore seek the advice of their doctor before undertaking any weight loss program.

None of the original statements or claims in this book have been examined or endorsed by the US Food and Drug Administration.

✂ *Introduction* ✂

For more than two decades, I have traveled all over the world communicating a simple message: *The quality of your health and even the length of your life will depend not so much on what your doctor does for you - despite all the major advances in the sick-care system - but on what you do for yourself between your doctor's visits.* This is nowhere more true than in the area of Weight Management. Therefore, this issue deserves to be front and center as we enter the new Wellness Revolution - the public groundswell in the industrialized world that is taking responsibility for optimizing health and celebrating life in the 21st Century.

Wellness and weight are two important contemporary concerns that you can only ignore at your own peril. They necessarily go together, but they are almost inversely related. You cannot focus on either one and neglect the other, because wellness is unattainable if your weight is unmanageable. If you starve yourself on any diet, your weight will certainly go down - but only at the expense of your wellness. That would *not* be a healthy solution. This book could be just the right alternative.

It is difficult to enjoy the best of health without the control of your weight - especially in this toxic American environment. Your weight could easily get out of control when fast and convenient junk food is everywhere, when technology has made us less dependent on physical exercise, and when entertainers will *make your day*, everyday, while you sit back in sedentary comfort to enjoy. These poor lifestyle habits could take a toll on the way you feel, the way you look, and most importantly, on the state of your health.

For many Americans, attainment of the 'body beautiful' is an all-important goal and yet it is both misleading and frustrating. It is misleading because your appearance is in no way as important as your health, and it is frustrating because if you have a weight issue, your best efforts have more than likely afforded you little long-term results.

However, dieting has become an American pastime. Fashion magazines, television infomercials and a host of weight loss gurus all make sure of that. So each year, millions decide its time to act. They resolve to lose some weight and their first choice is to go on a diet. But sooner or later, for most who manage to lose a significant amount, they begin to feel lethargic and miserable, and they give up in defeat. Many find that initial results are only temporary and they resign with disappointment as the weight comes right back.

It is no surprise then that the weight loss *industry* has become just that - an industry, a multibillion dollar recycling industry. But for the person who has the most difficult time controlling their weight, that is no comfort. For them, effective weight loss remains a personal problem. If that's you, then this book will be just what the name implies - a *solution*, a comprehensive and practical solution. It will show you a proven method to lose the extra pounds that you struggle with, even while you enjoy renewed energy and vitality.

If you could lose just five or ten percent of your present weight and keep it off, just imagine how you would look and how you would feel. But far more importantly, just imagine how much healthier your future would be. You have so much to gain and nothing to lose but those stubborn, unwanted pounds.

But the question arises, where do you begin? This whole area of diets and dieting has become so confused by the myriad of false ideas, fad products, fanciful gimmicks and some far-out, exaggerated claims for all three. There is so much misinformation and misrepresentation in the field. The sheer volume of diet books and programs, accompanied by all the celebrity endorsements and media hype, makes it almost impossible for you to make a rational decision about what kind of diet or weight loss program you should follow. You may be as confused as even the so-called experts are. But don't despair. This book will clearly show you how to lose weight effectively, while simultaneously improving your health and wellbeing.

Read on, there's hope!

The Enzyme Diet™ Solution faces the problem of weight management head-on. In **Part 1**, we look at **the Problem**. We must first understand why so many people keep fighting a losing battle and why it really matters that they're not losing weight. Ours is the fat generation and we are paying big-time in some major health consequences, outlined in Chapter 1. Despite all the many and varied weight loss programs and products which are selectively and critically reviewed in Chapter 2, the remedy for overweight and obesity remains elusive.

Most diets that restrict calories will yield some early results based on the simple energy (calorie) balance equation. To put it simply, if you avoid extra calories, you will initially lose extra weight. But the result is typically short term. During this semi-starvation mode, the body senses the dietary lack and reduces its metabolism accordingly. This works against the dieter and soon, even with reduced caloric input, the body continues to store fat and the losing trend is reversed. Hence, we see the common yo-yo dieting experience which is a real problem. Add to that, the fact that essential nutrients and enzymes are often lacking in the low calorie diets, so the cells become starved and the dieter experiences the early symptoms of inadequate nutrition. That exaggerates the problem.

People with weight challenges are often quick to blame everything and everyone but themselves. In Chapter 3, we get to the crux of the problem which goes beyond just calories. Surely, your genes are important but obviously, not deterministic. Of course hormones play a role, especially in women, but despite all the popular claims, neither insulin, thyroxine, estrogen, leptin nor all the other hormones being pursued can be condemned as the real culprit. Obesity is a truly multi-factoral condition, but lifestyle choices do play a very important role. The good news is that you can affect your net outcome by cultivating healthy habits, especially with the kind of ideal weight loss diet outlined at the end of the first major section.

That leads us to **the Solution** which is the focus of **Part II** in the book. First, we go back to basics in Chapter 4 to underscore the indispensable role of enzymes which are the neglected stars of the entire nutrition and metabolism performance. A new awareness of the essence of life and the important Food Enzyme Concept will teach you how to put enzymes to work for you. Enzymes are more than ordinary chemicals. They are biological molecules with destiny. Therefore, you will learn how to spare your enzyme potential so that you function at your physiological best. Of special importance, is the value of enzymes in helping to maintain your metabolism during weight loss.

The second major innovation is derived from a new approach to practical nutrition, which emphasizes the Seven Steps of Nutrition that result in exactly what your *cells* eat. This led to the development of the only guaranteed nutrient delivery system in the world. The details are laid out in Chapter 5, and for those who really want to know, the science behind it all is explained in an Appendix.

Putting it all together in Chapter 6, *The Enzyme Diet*™ is presented as a new alternative for effective weight loss that stays lost. This state-of-the-art meal replacement was fifteen years in design and development. It is packed with plant enzymes and contains all the essential nutrients to support your metabolism. It is low in calories and combined with a sensible dinner menu and vegetable/fruit snacks, provides adequate nutrition to feed your body. You can therefore lose weight consistently and yet feel invigorated and refreshed. It can otherwise serve as a Superfood supplement to the regular diet of those individuals simply in search of better health and wellness.

If you have no interest in the background to weight loss and the foundations of The Enzyme Diet™ Solution, you can go directly to this alternative starting point on Page 141.

You will be encouraged to make **your personal Application** of *The Enzyme Diet™ Solution* in the final **Part III** of the book. You will first learn to master the cycle of success in Chapter 7 that will allow you to avoid the most common dieting mistakes. The program is **as easy as 1-2-3** and **as simple as A-B-C**. It is complete with suggestions to get you started and tips to maximize your results, including an exit strategy. You will find this program entirely user-friendly and you will quickly frame a unique winning plan for yourself.

The essential principles of balanced nutrition are outlined in

Chapter 8 to allow you to devise your own menu to complement *The Enzyme Diet™*. Many practical ideas are included along with a variety of sensible dinner recipes, snacking tips and suggestions for maintaining your discipline when eating out. You will learn to eat right and that will make you feel right.

No diet program is complete without some emphasis on exercise. This is more important in the maintenance phase, but cardiovascular workouts and resistance (strength) training are important lifestyle habits to cultivate from the outset. To do both safely and efficiently will go a long way in maintaining your weight loss and making your weight management a lifelong behavioral style. Again, an original **1-2-3 approach** outlined in Chapter 9 will enable you to do just that.

By the time you get to the final Chapter, 10, you will have a new understanding of your weight problem and a handle on an effective, comprehensive solution - *The Enzyme Diet™ Solution*. You will realize that it is more than just another diet. It defines a fresh perspective that will sustain a new, responsible lifestyle. After reading this book, you will think differently and appreciate even more the value of feeding your cells and maintaining your metabolism, while losing your unwanted pounds. With such sensible and adequate nutrition, and a complementary exercise program, you will soon see the weight scale dropping and your health soaring. You will discover an amazing new wonderful You that enjoys a healthy and vibrant lifestyle which you will want to engage for a lifetime. You will celebrate life!

I hope you enjoy reading *The Enzyme Diet™ Solution* and then experience results similar to the many thousands who have already discovered that finally, there is a healthy way to effective weight loss that stays lost.

Congratulations, in advance!

Dr. Allan Somersall
Spring 2003

Part I

❧

Your Stubborn Weight
PROBLEM

Are You Fighting A Losing Battle?

❧ *Chapter 1* ❧

THE SILENT EPIDEMIC
The Fat Generation - Does It Really Matter?

Body weight is an intensely personal thing. There's no escaping it. It greets you every morning in the bathroom mirror, it follows you throughout the day by the reflections in the eyes of everyone you meet, and it whispers a 'good night' benediction as you put out your vanity light. It is your second face.

In every social setting, your appearance speaks volumes. Before you open your mouth, each extra pound communicates a silent message. As you speak, your visible weight provides a physical frame for all that you have to say. And after you depart from each encounter, your silhouette provides a personal echo that impresses upon the minds of others an indelible physical identity that makes for a gross caricature.

Overweight is a real emotional challenge. However you rationalize your own perception of self, you have no control over the perceptions of others, but can only speculate how and why they assess your lifestyle above your genes. You earn no social favors.

I suspect your sensitivity. Your apprehension is understandable and ever so natural. Weight distribution is the key, you say. But is it? Are you looking for assets and finding them in all the wrong places? And are you disappointed for all the wrong reasons?

It's no consolation, but the fact is that in today's America, you're clearly not alone. And you're also not alone in trying to do something about your presentation of self, only to be frustrated by no lasting results. More of you keeps coming back. And yet, there is still a bigger issue.

If you were asked to list the key factors in determining the quality of life and more particularly, the risks to avoidable illness and even premature death, what would immediately come to mind? Perhaps you might think of smoking or AIDS, or you might consider pollution or cholesterol. If you are a typical North American, you would probably miss the boat. You would not likely recognize the implications of the nation's silent epidemic. Yet, it's really no surprise. The Surgeon General pointed out as the new millenium dawned, that '*overweight and obesity may soon overtake tobacco as the leading cause of preventable deaths*' in the United States (1).

As a nation, we are now facing a growing weight crisis.

A National Crisis of Weighty Proportions

Yes, overweight is more than an aesthetic problem. It is not just a passing fad or a fashion statement. It is a real concern of most doctors because it does have dire consequences. Yet, there is no doubt whatsoever that it has become a growing epidemic in our generation. To illustrate this, just consider these pertinent facts (1):

    ◆ A whopping **61% of adults** in the United States - 120 million of us - are now considered to be overweight, including 26% who are even clinically obese. Don't be confused, we will define these different terms later. That first shocking number has been growing steadily over four decades. It reflects our way of life. *We're the most affluent country on earth but we're also the most overweight.* That is more than embarrassing. Something must be fundamentally wrong in our culture.

    ◆ Would you have guessed that **300,000 deaths** each year in the United States are associated with obesity? Compare this with the 400,000 who die prematurely from cigarette smoking. But note the important contrast: *smoking is on the decline while obesity is on the rise.* Let's put this in perspective. This is eight times the number who die from AIDS, and more than the combined total of all who die from alcohol, drugs, firearms and motor vehicle accidents put together. That's newsworthy.

    ◆ There are at least **30 serious chronic medical condi-**

tions affected by obesity. These include heart disease, certain types of cancer, Type II diabetes, stroke, arthritis, breathing problems, and psychological disorders such as depression. That should certainly make you stop and think.

♦ Imagine that **13% of children** aged 6-11 years and 14% of *adolescents* aged 12-19 years are already overweight. This prevalence has almost tripled for adolescents in the past two decades. We also know that overweight children are more prone to develop adult obesity. So much for the future trends. Parents need to take responsibility early, but the external pressures to influence young lifestyles are winning the day.

♦ The Center for Disease Control (CDC) in Atlanta published a recent survey of four key lifestyle areas for all Americans (2). The findings are revealing of **our delinquent choices**:

- 23% eat enough fruits and vegetables
- 26% engage in regular physical leisure activity
- 38% have healthy weights
- 72% are non smokers, and worst of all, only
- 3% engage in all four healthy practices.

♦ The increases in overweight and obesity cut across all ages, racial and ethnic groups, and both genders. Socioeconomic factors do have some influences but the epidemic is widespread, **crossing all demographic lines.**

♦ The total direct and indirect economic cost of overweight and obesity in the United States was about **$117 billion** in the year 2000. That alone should get the entire nation's attention. The direct healthcare costs refer to preventive, diagnostic and treatment services to obese people. This would include, for example, physician visits, medications, hospital and nursing home care. Together, weight issues consume about 6% of the total health expenditure in the United States. Indirect costs of overweight and obesity include the value of wages lost by people unable to work because of resulting illness or disability, as well as the value of future earnings lost by premature death. This total economic cost is *comparable to the costs of cigarette smoking.*

These facts and many more reveal the high prevalence of overweight and obesity in the United States. It is a sobering reminder of the dark side of prosperity and the changes brought about by the industrial and technological advances of the last century. No matter how you look at sample statistics like these, the reality is clear that we have become, by and large, a fat generation. **For the first time in American history, a majority of adults are now considered overweight**. In fact, clinical obesity increased by 50% between 1980 and 1994. That is a true epidemic, except that it is not exactly a contagious condition. It is a cultural phenomenon, reflecting both individual predisposition and inappropriate response to a toxic lifestyle environment. We are indeed facing a real national crisis of weighty proportions.

'The Enzyme Diet™ Solution' is addressed *personally* to you, but it is our hope that in the course of time, this book will help point America in the right direction. However, as we get started, we should first pay attention to the underlying causes of the growing epidemic.

ॐ

Causes Of This Growing Epidemic

When global trends are apparent, it is unlikely that any single person can shoulder the complete blame. Clearly, for each individual body weight will be the result of a combination of many factors and influences. These must include genetic, metabolic, emotional, behavioral, environmental, cultural and socioeconomic considerations. Such multifactoral conditions should always make us slow to judge or condemn any person before we know all the facts that determine how truly challenged they are. Unfortunately, in our culture, discrimination and mistreatment of persons with obesity is widespread and often considered socially acceptable. Even less overweight individuals can become victims of derogatory jokes and embarrassing innuendo among the family, on the job or at different social gatherings. Of course, behavioral changes can and often do make a big difference, but there's so much more to consider.

Scientists have suspected for a long time that there are dozens, if not hundreds of genes and associated hormones that regulate the ***energy (calorie) balance equation***. That's the essential relationship between our energy input and output, leaving the net balance for storage as fat. We'll discuss that in detail later in Chapter 3. For now, we simply observe that this complex array of inherited factors remains elusive. It no doubt contributes to the predisposition of some individuals to put on more than their fair share of body weight. Obesity for some is a chronic condition with a strong familial component. It's a battle they may even feel destined to lose. Some people protest that they sometimes only 'look at food' and that's enough to add a few pounds to their already embarrassing frame. But as Shakespeare would say, '*methinks they doth protest too much*.' It's not deterministic and it does not let anyone off the hook. After all, mere genes could not make anyone fat. They merely set up a susceptibility to gaining weight under certain conditions.

Sure we can point a finger at someone we know who spends too much time in front of their computer or watching the wide world of sports from their comfortable sofa, while nibbling all the time. Someone else may be too gluttonous or just addicted to french fries or soda. But such individual answers would be too simplistic to account for such a widespread epidemic. After all, **the whole nation's waistline is bulging.**

It is a known fact that the American diet has changed drastically in our generation. We live in a land of plenty - but that's not the real issue here. Our farmers produce plenty of fiber-rich grains and cereals, and our markets abound in raw fruits and vegetables. Unfortunately however, that's not our first preference in the fast-paced, industrialized society we live in. Driven by convenience and gullible to the effective marketing appeals to taste, sight and smell, we have become victims to the fast convenience food, processed food and even junk food industries. How could we resist the saturation advertising of these marketing wizards when the food industry spends about $10 billion a year on advertising? McDonalds alone spends more than $1 billion and Coca Cola more than $800 million to get their message across.

We have become satisfied consumers of unhealthy, high-calorie foods which we swallow in larger quantities and in less time. We eat out far more and take out our favorite fast foods from some 170,000 available restaurants across the nation. For the even more sedentary, we order over the phone for fast guaranteed delivery. No sweat. No hassle. And for all this, we pay a big price.

Over the last two decades, caloric intake in the United States has risen nearly 10% for men and 7% for women. **Modern diets are exploding with fat and sugar.** Although low fat alternatives in supermarkets and some restaurants have capped the unhealthy splurge, fat is still everywhere. Today, we still take in 35% of calories as fat. This is a downward trend compared to the 40% in 1990. But the best advice from professionals such as the American Heart Association would be to limit us even more, to just 30% of calories as fat.

In addition to the sugars that occur naturally in foods, the average American diet now includes 20 teaspoons of added refined sugar a day, much of that in soft drinks and prepared foods. That's all empty calories. It's an energy burden with no other nutritional benefit. If there's no benefit, why do we consume so much sugar? Animal studies have demonstrated a different kind of benefit. Researchers at the University of Minnesota's Obesity Center, monitored the impact sugar has on mood-enhancing circuits in the brain. To put it simply, sugar gives rats - and by extension, humans - a buzz. We are programmed to pamper our sweet tooth because it tastes *oh, so good* and we feel *oh, so fine*. However, in a smaller study, Danish scientists demonstrated the negative impact of sugar on body weight. These scientists compared the weight changes of overweight middle-aged people using either table sugar (sucrose) or artificial sweetener with little or no calories. The former gained while the latter lost, underlining the fact that sugar in the diet is an important factor in pushing up our weight.

But let's not be too quick to blame everything on the fat and sugar we consume. **We're guilty of simply eating too much - period!** Too much of everything.

In an industry where cost of goods is not compelling and competition is fierce, portion sizes have increased across the board. Most restaurant portions today are twice as large as a standard serving. In fact, *two could often eat for the price of one.* But consumers have now come to anticipate these large portions and 'regular' sizes seem somewhat skimpy. According to the US Department of Agriculture, the number of total calories available in the food we consume has gone up drastically, by about 300 calories per person per day, over the past 30 years (6). We also burn 260 less calories each day, on average. That single observation alone could explain the obesity epidemic. The typical adult diet has gone up by so many calories per day, that if not offset by metabolism and exercise, it could theoretically add some 30 pounds per person per year. That ought to set off the alarm, and it has to some limited degree. A recent survey by the American Dietetic Association found that 40% of Americans claim that they are taking more care in selecting what they eat in order to achieve balanced nutrition and a healthy diet. That's trending positively upward. Those who were not, confessed to not working 'to give up the foods they like,' and to be 'satisfied' with the way they currently eat.

But intake is only one side of the equation. What about burning off the excess calories?

Here again, we're moving as a nation in the wrong direction. Exercise and sports have become huge industries but primarily on television. Millions are content to just sit and watch the superstars earn their astronomic salaries having fun, playing games they love. But their fans suffer in armchairs. **In a nation so obsessed with sports, we are dying for lack of physical activity**. What a paradox!

Only 22% of adult Americans get the recommended amount of regular physical activity of *any* intensity during leisure time. This should be done at least four or five times a week for at least 20 to 30 minutes. About 15% get the recommended amount of vigorous activity, that is, three times a week for at least 20 minutes. As much as 25% of adults actually claim to do *no* physical activity at all in their leisure time (3).

Technology has made transportation and even domestic chores most convenient and affordable. We even use remote controls to avoid walking across the room. Few would choose to climb a flight of stairs or two, when an escalator or elevator will do. The internet and e-commerce have now revolutionized the way we live and the effect is to make yet more couch-potatoes.

Adults are still free agents, at least in America. We can overeat and vegetate, and consequently gain weight, if we want to. However, what is even more disturbing about this far-too-common lifestyle is that we are unwittingly perhaps, and in a myriad of ways, passing on the same unhealthy tendencies to the next generation. Many children and young people are being raised by neglect on a diet of fast, convenience and junk foods. Their generation is falling victim as they substitute video games for vigorous athletics and sports. More than 40% of adolescents watch more than two hours of television each day, a known correlate with overweight and obesity. They have forgotten the great outdoors. Physical education *classes* are disappearing all across America. Only about 25% of young people, between 12-21 years of age, actually participate in light to moderate activity like walking, swimming or cycling on a daily basis. About 50% regularly engage in vigorous physical activity, whereas about 25% report no vigorous physical activity and 14% report no recent vigorous or light to moderate activity.

We may indeed have become 'the most sedentary generation of people in the history of the world'. Yet, we know that in addition to helping to control weight, physical activity decreases the risk of dying from coronary heart disease and reduces the risk of developing diabetes, hypertension and perhaps colon and breast cancer.

Putting it all together, the consumption of **too many empty calories** and the practice of **too little exercise** combine in endemic proportions to increase the storage of the **excess as fat**, leading to the obesity epidemic. That has now become a true 'crisis'.

Predictably, that's not without consequences.

Beware of Health Consequences

Obesity has consequences. Some of these are only superficial. It's the awareness that clothes no longer fit; or that the 'eyes' on the beach connote a different message; or that becoming the subject of innuendo or party jokes feels disconcerting; or that reading fashion magazines seems more depressing than entertaining. Realities like these drive millions to weight-loss programs of all types and descriptions. Shedding those extra pounds, losing a size or two in clothes, or just an inch or two here or there, become at first a playful fantasy, then a passion and often a program of desperation. People want to look better and to feel better.

Unfortunately though, those who need to lose weight *less* are very often, the ones more committed and desperate. On the other hand, those who need to lose weight *more*, are sometimes less disturbed and tend rather to become insecure, frustrated and disillusioned to the point of indifference. But for these latter individuals, the consequences could be more severe. They go beyond mere appearance to threaten the maintenance of good health, to impact the course of chronic disease and often to contribute to premature death. Most studies have shown an increase in mortality rate associated with obesity. In fact, obese individuals actually have a 50-100% increased risk of death from all causes, compared with normal weight individuals. Most of this increased risk is due to cardiovascular causes.

The primary concern with overweight and obesity must therefore be one of health and not appearance. This is not a Hollywood creation. It is a real issue of everyday life where the weight issue becomes a health concern. As a doctor, sometimes I wish I could impress this more on patients so that they would get off the message of popular magazines and talk shows. They need to hear the real truth about their bodies and their clinical prognosis for the future.

If you face a weight challenge, it would do you well to hear, loud and clear, the **health warning**, first and foremost. Beyond that, you are free to cater to your appearance and to fashion as your own personality dictates. Lose those extra few pounds to make you look and feel good. But make no mistake about it, as someone said *'when you have your health, you have almost everything.'* Likewise, when you lose it, you also lose almost everything. Therefore, health considerations are paramount when you consider your weight. You should become an avid health-watcher.

TABLE 1 on the following pages, summarizes the major health consequences of overweight and obesity. The message is clear. However, take note at the same time, that a modest weight loss of 5 to 15% of total body weight in a person who is overweight or obese, can reduce the risk factors for some important diseases, particularly heart disease. It can lower blood pressure, lower blood sugar and improve cholesterol levels. The benefit is more pronounced for anyone with other health risk factors, such as hypertension, elevated cholesterol, smoking, diabetes, a sedentary lifestyle, a personal and/or family history of heart disease and some forms of cancer.

It is now very obvious that weight is a major health challenge. So, what's the solution? You must take control.

Table 1.

Health Consequences Of Overweight and Obesity

PREMATURE DEATH
· An estimated 300,000 deaths per year may be attributed to obesity.
· The risk of death rises with increasing weight.
· Even moderate weight excess (10 to 20 pounds for a person of average height) increases the risk of death, particularly among adults 30 to 64 years.
· Individuals who are obese (BMI >30)*have a 50 to 100% increased risk of premature death from all causes, compared to individuals with a healthy weight.

HEART DISEASE
· The incidence of heart disease (heart attack, congestive heart failure, sudden cardiac death, angina or chest pain, and abnormal heart rhythm) is increased in persons who are overweight or obese (BMI>25).*
· High blood pressure is twice as common in adults who are obese than in those who are at a healthy weight.
· Obesity is associated with elevated triglycerides (blood fat) and decreased HDL cholesterol ("good cholesterol").

DIABETES
· A weight gain of 11 to 18 pounds increases a person's risk of developing type 2 diabetes to twice that of individuals who have not gained weight.
· Over 80% of people with diabetes are overweight or obese.

CANCER
· Overweight and obesity are associated with an increased risk for some types of cancer including endometrial (cancer of the lining of the uterus), colon, gall bladder, prostate, kidney, and postmenopausal breast cancer.
· Women gaining more than 20 pounds from age 18 to midlife double their risk of postmenopausal breast cancer, compared to women whose weight remains stable.

BREATHING PROBLEMS
· Sleep apnea (interrupted breathing while sleeping) is more common in obese persons.
· Obesity is associated with a higher prevalence of asthma.

Table 1 cont'd

ARTHRITIS
· For every 2-pound increase in weight, the risk of developing arthritis is increased by 9 to 13%.
· Symptoms of arthritis can improve with weight loss.

REPRODUCTIVE COMPLICATIONS

· Complications of pregnancy

· Obesity during pregnancy is associated with increased risk of death in both the baby and the mother and increases the risk of maternal high blood pressure by 10 times.
· In addition to many other complications, women who are obese during pregnancy are more likely to have gestational diabetes and problems with labor and delivery.
· Infants born to women who are obese during pregnancy are more likely to be high birth weight and, therefore, may face a higher rate of Cesarean section delivery and low blood sugar (which can be associated with brain damage and seizures).
· Obesity during pregnancy is associated with an increased risk of birth defects, particularly neural tube defects, such as spina bifida.

· Obesity in premenopausal women is associated with irregular menstrual cycles and infertility.

ADDITIONAL HEALTH CONSEQUENCES
· Overweight and obesity are associated with increased risks of gall bladder disease, incontinence, increased surgical risk, and depression.
· Obesity can affect the quality of life through limited mobility and decreased physical endurance as well as through social, academic and job discrimination.

* BMI will be discussed later in this chapter, p. 22

Ref. US Surgeon General's Report (1)

Take Control Of Your Future

If you're overweight or obese, *your weight could make you sick.* We've heard that same mantra for decades. The alarm has been sounding in many quarters because of the obvious consequences. And almost all health experts advocate the same general approach.

In principle, these traditional weight loss professionals tell us that it all comes down to a simple formula: *eat less calories and exercise more.* But that is a gross over- simplification and in practice, the vast majority of dieters who attempt to lose weight soon discover that their early success is only frustrated by subsequent failure. In the medium to long term, their weight returns, and often with a vengeance. The net result is that since the 1950's, despite all the advice and the plethora of weight loss diets, the rate of obesity has tripled. We've been losing this battle again and again.

Here's another paradox. People who are overweight often go on some sort of 'diet', attempting to reduce their caloric *intake* to the same level of their caloric use or below. Unfortunately, this is physiologically difficult. Why? Because they typically have such an abnormally low caloric use associated with their sedentary lifestyles, that to achieve their goal, they need a kind of 'starvation diet'. This must of necessity be short-lived. That is why **95% of Americans who attempt to achieve a healthy body weight by dieting alone, fail.**

Yet Americans are persuaded that weight loss is a worthwhile goal and are willing to spend big in pursuit of a more normal appearance. It is estimated that some 50 million Americans or more enroll each year in some kind of weight-loss program involving special diet regimens, under medical or some other supervision. Many others go-it-alone with their own diets, following any of the myriad that are always available on the market. Driven more by fashion and advertising than by health con-siderations, they put out over $34 billion each year on weight loss prod-ucts and services. This expenditure would include consumer dollars spent on all the many and varied weight loss or weight maintenance strategies. These include low calorie foods, artificially sweetened prod-ucts such as diet sodas, memberships of commercial weight-loss centers and a host of fad diet products. The success rates are ubiquitously low, but the demand persists and the promise of each new offering keeps hope alive and captivates a following.

When all else fails, some people become desperate. They are driven to extreme measures like stomach stapling (gastric bypass or gastroplasty) to curb consumption, or to liposuction to remove the excess fat already there. The latter is a risky invasive surgical procedure which quite literally vacuums fat from under the skin in areas that bulge or sag. In 1998, there were some 400,000 liposuctions and about 60,000 gastric bypass procedures carried out in the United States. These are crude, impractical and often ineffective stop-gap solutions that fail to deal with the fundamental problem. They should be reserved for the most 'hopelessly obese' cases. More normal individuals must find a better solution to their weight problem.

That's where you come in. You must take control of your future. You need to find a solution that works for you. And rest assured, there is one.

We'll discuss all this in much more practical detail throughout the book, but suffice it to say here that weight control must be a life-long affair. In real terms, all the relevant factors such as lifestyle, diet, exercise and physiology must converge for permanent success. It's a weight *management* issue. If you just hang in there, perhaps **The Enzyme Diet™** might be the exact **solution** you've been looking for.

Basic Concepts of Weight Management

Before we get ahead of ourselves, let's get back to the basics. What exactly are we talking about? Who is overweight? What is obesity? How can these be measured reliably? You should first want to be clear how you fit into this picture and what exactly you ought to be concerned about. The answers might surprise you.

Defining the Terms

'*Overweight*' refers generally to an excess of body weight compard to set standards. But the excess weight may come from either muscle, bone, fat and/or body water. *'Obesity'* refers more significantly to having an abnormally high proportion of body fat. Thus, you can be overweight without being obese, if you are for example, an athlete or bodybuilder with a lot of lean muscle. Chances are though, that if you are significantly overweight, you would tend to be also obese. However, in quantitative terms, the term 'obese' is usually reserved for the higher end of overweight people. Interestingly, the prevalence of overweight is higher for men than women but conversely, the prevalence of obesity is higher for women than men. Both parameters can be determined by using different methods.

The most common standardization parameter used today involves what is known as the Body Mass Index (BMI).

i.   *Body Mass Index*

Most professionals today consider this the measurement of choice in the area of body weight as it relates to health. An expert panel, convened by the US National Institute of Health (NIH) in 1998, recommended that the Body Mass Index (BMI) be used to formally classify overweight and obesity. Your BMI is a number derived from a quick and simple calculation, based on your height and weight. It is applicable to both males and females and it can be conveniently used as a standardized measure for both 'overweight' and 'obesity' in adults.

The formula for calculating your BMI is simply to divide your weight in kilograms by your height in meters squared. When using pounds and inches, the revision calls for you to multiply your weight in pounds by 700 and then dividing the result by your height in inches squared. (This is a close approximation used by the American Dietetic Association. The National Institute of Health, (NIH) uses the more precise conversion factor of 704.5).

$$\text{BMI} = \frac{\text{wt (kg)}}{\text{Height squared (m}^2)} \quad \text{or} \quad \frac{\text{wt (lbs) x 700}}{\text{Height squared (in}^2)}$$

For the reader who could not be bothered, **Table 2** is a reference chart that allows you to simply read off your BMI (4). First, find your height (in inches) in the left vertical column, and then go across that row to find your body weight (in pounds), then the actual number at the very top of that column is your BMI.

Most professionals accept the term 'overweight' to apply to those with a BMI between 25 and 30 kg/m², and consider 'obese' to refer to those with a BMI of 30 kg/m² or higher, even though the two terms are not mutually exclusive (since obese persons are also overweight).

Table 2

Body Mass Index Chart

Height (inches)	19	20	21	22	23	24	25	26	27	28	29	30	31	32	33	34	35
								Body Weight (pounds)									
58	91	96	100	105	110	115	119	124	129	134	138	143	148	153	158	162	167
59	94	99	104	109	114	119	124	128	133	138	143	148	153	158	163	168	173
60	97	102	107	112	118	123	128	133	138	143	148	153	158	163	168	174	179
61	100	106	111	116	122	127	132	137	143	148	153	158	164	169	174	180	185
62	104	109	115	120	126	131	136	142	147	153	158	164	169	175	180	186	191
63	107	113	118	124	130	135	141	146	152	158	163	169	175	180	186	191	197
64	110	116	122	128	134	140	145	151	157	163	169	174	180	186	192	197	204
65	114	120	126	132	138	144	150	156	162	168	174	180	186	192	198	204	210
66	118	124	130	136	142	148	155	161	167	173	179	186	192	198	204	210	216
67	121	127	134	140	146	153	159	166	172	178	185	191	198	204	211	217	223
68	125	131	138	144	151	158	164	171	177	184	190	197	203	210	216	223	230
69	128	135	142	149	155	162	169	176	182	189	196	203	209	216	223	230	236
70	132	139	146	153	160	167	174	181	188	195	202	209	216	222	229	236	243
71	136	143	150	157	165	172	179	186	193	200	208	215	222	229	236	243	250
72	140	147	154	162	169	177	184	191	199	206	213	221	228	235	242	250	258
73	144	151	159	166	174	182	189	197	204	212	219	227	235	242	250	257	265
74	148	155	163	171	179	186	194	202	210	218	225	233	241	249	256	264	272
75	152	160	168	176	184	192	200	208	216	224	232	240	248	256	264	272	279
76	156	164	172	180	189	197	205	213	221	230	238	246	254	263	271	279	287

The limitation of the BMI is that it does not do justice to very muscular people who may fall into the 'overweight' category while they are indeed quite healthy and fit. After all, who would choose to label someone like the NBA superstar Shaquille O'Neal as overweight? On the other extreme, some unfortunate people who have lost muscle mass, such as the elderly, diseased or even malnourished, may fall into the 'healthy weight' designation using BMI, while they may be suffering from under-lying illness or have reduced nutritional reserves. In other words, BMI does not tell the whole story, even though it is very useful as a general guideline to monitor trends in the population, or for individuals who do not fall into exceptional categories. In simple terms, BMI correlates well with total body fat for the vast majority of people.

What is your BMI? Take a moment to do the calculation just now, or even read it off the chart in Table 2. Are you overweight or 'obese'? If so, this book has some great news for you. If your BMI is greater that 25, you must think of health risks. The greater your BMI in fact, the higher your risk. It is simply prudent to consider a sensible weight loss program that will work for you. If you have a BMI below 25 kg/m^2, you may still be interested in losing a few pounds for your own personal reasons. You'll look better and feel better and perhaps, get back into your favorite clothes. That's reason enough, but whatever your reason for wanting to lose weight, **The Enzyme Diet™ Solution** will guide you to a healthy way to achieve your goal. You will learn how to lose weight effectively, while feeling great, and also learn how to keep it off.

The actual *distribution of body fat* tells us more. In general terms, increased abdominal or upper body fat - as reflected in larger waistlines, paunches, middle age spread, pot bellies or 'beer bellies' - is related to increased risk of developing heart disease, diabetes, high blood pressure, gallbladder disease, stroke and certain cancers. It is in fact, associated with overall mortality (the likelihood of death). Women with waistlines measuring more than 35 inches, and men whose waists exceed 40 inches may, in either case, be at particular risk for developing health problems. People with this type of fat distribution are now commonly referred to as 'apples'. The good news is that this type of fat is more sus-ceptible to weight loss. It tends to come and go more easily. Sensible dieting and moderate exercise make a big difference for these individu-als.

In contrast, when body fat is concentrated in the lower body -

around the hips, for example - it may be somewhat less harmful in terms of the likelihood of disease and potential mortality. People with this type of fat distribution are similarly identified as 'pears'. The bad news is that 'pears' tend to have more stubborn fat. But with a good dietary and exercise program, effective weight loss can still be achieved.

Unfortunately however, there truly is no consolation for either 'apples' or 'pears'. If you have excess weight to contend with, you have an increased health risk to deal with. Weight loss should therefore be a priority in either case.

ii.   *Metabolic Syndrome*

We now appreciate that obesity ought not to be considered in isolation. In fact, it is commonly associated with a complex of other conditions including high blood pressure, poor cholesterol profiles (high triglycerides and/or low HDL) and high blood sugar. This complex of symptoms and signs together constitute the so-called 'metabolic syndrome' which has been recognized since the 1920's. The name itself is misleading since one's metabolism need not be defective. It is more likely a multi-factoral phenomenon in which genes and lifestyle factors all play significant roles.

A recent study estimated that at least 47 million American adults suffer from this syndrome. It greatly increases the risk of diabetes, heart disease and stroke. The National Institute of Health (NIH) has formulated a definition to include those patients with three or more of the following:

- A waist of at least 40 inches in men and 35 inches in women;
- Circulating fat (triglycerides) exceeding 150 mg/dl;
- HDL levels less than 40 mgs in men and 50 mgs in women;
- Blood pressure of at least 135/80; and
- Blood sugar of at least 110 mg/dl

The syndrome clearly is prevalent and is tending to increase with adult years. This is one syndrome however, that is exquisitely lifestyle-sensitive. If those people affected would only pay attention and respond by appropriate lifestyle interventions, the results could be dramatic in both quality and quantity of life.

Could that be you? It's time for action.

Your Call To Action

Overweight and obesity have been a neglected public health problem for far too long. This has led to irresponsibility on the part of many individuals. There has also been a lack of structural and institutional restraints that have created an environment where the path of least resistance clearly leads to unhealthy food indulgence and increasingly sedentary lifestyles. This starts at an early age and there is no apparent end in sight.

In the face of such an epidemic with its major potential health and economic consequences, something must be done. On December 13, 2001 the US Federal Government released a tough, hard-hitting report we referred to earlier, entitled *"The Surgeon General's Call to Action to Prevent and Decrease Overweight and Obesity."* (1) It was a rallying cry, to do in this area what the Nixon administration attempted in its *War on Cancer* program more than three decades ago. Perhaps, an even more relevant analogy would be the attack on smoking that federal officials promoted with much success in the last decade. Obesity and smoking are both examples of essentially private, lifestyle issues. They both have strong health and economic considerations, and they both engage choices that highlight First Amendment privileges. Yet behavior modification still requires both private and public response, all based on good information and intelligent action.

The Surgeon General's Report therefore, was first designed to draw national attention to the serious health and economic implications of this growing problem and then to appeal for some fundamental changes at all levels.

The report called for the entire nation to take an informed, sensitive approach to communicate with and educate the American people primarily about the health issues related to overweight and obesity. Everyone must work together to change the perception of these conditions at all ages. There is a real need to educate healthcare providers and students in health professions about the prevention and treatment of weight disorders across the life span. Expectant mothers need to understand the many benefits of breastfeeding, one of which is to provide fewer empty calories and less overweight children. Schools and communities need appropriate education about healthy eating habits and regular physical activity at all ages. Most importantly, emphasis must be placed on **the role of the individual consumer** in making wise food choices and participation in regular exercise.

In the end, it comes down to the individual, just like you, taking responsibility and making the right choices. Lifestyle and behavior in a free society cannot be legislated or even dictated. It is up to you to become aware of your own weight status and its implications. Parents of course should consider the impact on their children and care givers must watch out for the elderly.

So, where do you stand? Again, **what is your BMI**? Is weight an issue for you? You may be concerned about your physical appearance and the negative stereotyping in the world of fashion and social interaction. That's good motivation to pay attention. You may recognize that the way you feel and your level of fitness is negatively influenced by some degree of extra weight that you would love to get rid of. Perhaps you can recall a slimmer, trimmer, fitter you that you felt much more comfortable with. You had more confidence, more energy and more resilience then.

Or, could it be that you are at increased risk of morbidity or illness just because of your overweight condition and you are constrained to do something about it. Your doctor keeps telling you that you should - you ought to - lose some weight for your own better health. Do you have other risk factors that compound the situation such as hypertension, diabetes, some lung disease, osteoarthritis, heart disease, or any of the other complicating conditions? Then **you must take action in your own self-defense.**

What do you have to lose? Perhaps nothing but weight - a little of it or a lot of it. This is a challenge for sure, but it's worth it. You already know that. This book will give you answers, and provide guidance and hope. **The Enzyme Diet™ Solution** could be just the thing you need.

If you've tried to lose weight before and failed, or if you've succeeded at first, only to regain the same relentless burden - take heart, for you are not alone! That is the ubiquitous pattern for millions like you. The next chapter will review some of the most popular weight loss programs and suggest some reasons why, together they represent **the elusive remedy.**

Maybe you'll discover **why your last diet probably failed.**

Chapter 2

THE ELUSIVE REMEDY
Your Last Diet - Did It Fail?

When it comes to weight management and the frustration of those who really struggle to gain control of their issues, you can be sure that you are not alone. That is the norm. It is for most, a losing battle.

Yet, some people it seems, are blessed with efficient metabolism just by their genetic inheritance. But that's not the real difference. Others find that fitness and exercise come easily to them and from their early childhood, they make that a lifestyle habit. But again, that's not the point. In a common environment, we are all making choices. Sooner or later, we must take responsibility for the way we choose to live. In the affluence of American society and culture, the quantity and quality of foods that we choose to eat are essentially a reflection of our values and our discipline. So is our sedentary lifestyle. Therefore, you cannot exempt your genes or your circumstances. It takes much more than that.

However, despite the poor track record for dieting, each year millions of Americans face themselves in the mirror and for one reason or another, they decide to lose some weight. Priority number one is always to focus on what they eat - to go on a diet of some kind that they hope will do the trick. No wonder then that at any given time, two in five women and one in four men in the United States are trying to lose weight. They resort to a variety of different methods, including limits to their diet, increased exercise, behavior modification, a handful of drugs and even surgery. But by far the largest group resorts to dieting - changing their eating habits - as the key to losing those undesirable pounds that affect their self image as much, if not more than their health. So again, you're really not alone.

In the Fall of 1997, representatives from the academic community, government, the weight loss industry and consumer advocacy groups all met in Washington, DC for a conference with the headline: *"Commercial Weight Loss Products and Programs - What Consumers Stand to Gain and Lose."* (1)   This was the first conference of its kind to bring together all the various parties and stakeholders in this growing multi-billion dollar industry.   In fact, it was now much more than just another industry, it had become a major public health issue.   Therefore, participants in this forum focused on the main challenge: *The Continuing Rise of Obesity in the United States*.   This conference was conceived as a coordinated effort by all concerned groups to better understand the problem of uncontrolled weight.   They sought to explore ways to improve the information that consumers routinely receive about the nature of obesity and weight loss products and programs.

In their summary, these front-line experts concluded that in spite of the widespread promotion and marketing of thousands of treatments, devices, therapies, programs and products that are supposed to induce weight loss and prevent regain, the most remarkable aspect of most of them is - you guessed it - their **failure** rate. As we pointed out in the last chapter, it is now common knowledge, that up to 95% of dieters have made little real progress in their weight and control of the same, when monitored a mere five years after their initial commitment. Much of the time, these desperate individuals give up in frustration. They tend to set unrealistic expectations while making inadequate lifestyle changes. Failure is therefore no surprise.

Despite advice of so many weight loss 'experts', many Americans are avoiding professionally supervised weight loss centers and are turning to fad-diet books, dietary supplements, internet offerings and do-it-yourself weight loss solutions.   They want a magic pill or a program that will help them to lose weight quickly and keep it off permanently.   There really is no such thing, but at least you should know what is available out there. Diets by the hundreds are popularized every year and dieters by the millions are misguided in their search.

Almost all the diets and diet programs out there are fundamentally designed to reduce the intake of calories. After all, what is labeled *the energy balance equation* or *the calorie balance equation* is generally acknowledged by all professionals. It tells us simply, you recall, that the difference between the input and the output of energy in the form of calories will be stored as fat. In reality, almost any low-calorie diet will result in initial weight loss and in addition, any diuretic effect that results in loss of water, will show on the weight scales as a further loss. However, what one must always be conscious of, is the indispensable need for adequate nutrition to feed the body and maintain metabolism. One must also avoid reducing muscle and other lean body mass.

Any low-calorie approach must consider the calorie sources in food. All food can be broken down into seven essential classes: protein, carbohydrates (starch and sugar), fats (including essential fatty acids), fiber (mostly indigestible bulk in the diet), vitamins, minerals and water. Only the first three of these provide sources of energy in the form of calories. The others are support players. Fat is by far the most calorie-dense, providing *nine* kilocalories per gram, whereas carbohydrate and proteins provide only *four* kilocalories per gram. We have not included another major culprit - alcohol - which itself provides *seven* kilocalories per gram. But then again, alcohol is not a food, although it often contributes significantly to caloric intake and must be considered in the overall picture, whenever it is consumed by those seeking to control their weight status.

For the purist reading this, a word of clarification is in order. A **calorie** is defined as the amount of energy required to raise the temperature of one gram of water by one degree centigrade. A **kilocalorie** is equal to 1000 calories, but in the field of food and nutrition the term 'calorie' is used as an abbreviation for a kilocalorie. It should technically be always written with a capital 'C' for distinction, but the popular use of 'calories' has made this common notation acceptable almost everywhere.

Getting back to diets and dieting, we will now briefly review some of the more important diets that have dominated the market. We will consider the various approaches in terms of how they focus on the sources of calories in the diet. Historically, the first attack was on *fat* in the diet, then a tolerance of high *protein* (associated with low carbohydrate) was advocated, and to complete the triad, the focus shifted to controlling *carbohydrates*. We'll begin this short selective review in that same order.

Note: You need not get bogged down with the wide variety of diets on the market today, unless you are really interested. You may choose to go directly to the type of diet that you have tried or

have been considering and then go on from there directly to the last section of the chapter on Meal Replacements (Page 57).

LOW FAT DIETS
Are Not Always The Answer

Since fat is the most calorie-rich food source and fat is the real enemy target in weight loss, it is not surprising that this approach would be first, front and center. Surprisingly though, the two leading diet programs in this group were not developed primarily as weight loss diets, but as part of a management program for cardiovascular disease. One came from a conscientious patient and the other from a competent physician.

The Pritikin Diet

In the late 1950's, Nathan Pritikin was diagnosed with heart disease. As a wise and responsible patient, he adopted a low-fat, high-fiber diet and began a moderate exercise program. His interventions proved pivotal. Subsequent medical examinations revealed dramatic improvements in his own health, which led him to develop the Pritikin Diet Program, essentially based on his personal experience.

He opened the first Pritikin Longevity Center in 1976 so that he could help others with similar medical problems restore their health. In effect, though, a distinct and lucrative side benefit of this lifestyle modification program was indeed weight-loss. The rest, it can be said, is history.

Today his son Robert is still aggressively leading the charge. He authored the more recent bestseller, *The Pritikin Principle* (Time Life, 2000) in which he advocated the same basic calorie density solution to weight loss. It puts a new spin on something that nutritionists have been preaching for many years. Some foods are richer in calories - that is more dense - and to effectively cut calories, it would make sense to reduce the more high-calorie or calorie-dense foods. Pritikin does the work for you by arranging foods according to calories per pound and then encourages the dieter to strike a balance of low and medium calorie-dense foods. The high calorie-dense foods are reserved for occasional indulgences only.

The Pritikin Diet is almost vegetarian. It encourages the consumption of large amounts of whole grains and vegetables. As such, it is very high in fiber, extremely low in total fat and saturated fat in particular, and low in cholesterol. Only 10-15% of total calories are derived from fat. The program also calls for regular exercise - at least 45 minutes of walking each day.

No one could argue with the health benefits of eating less fat and more whole grains, plus fresh fruits and vegetables. There is a vast body of scientific literature to demonstrate the value of this in the prevention of many degenerative diseases and it has become a recurring theme for nutritionists and dieticians. Clinical studies at the Pritikin Longevity Center's have shown that this diet, combined with a structured exercise program, does produce expected weight loss, at least in the short term, and it does lower cholesterol and triglyceride levels. High fiber foods provide bulk and in theory, help to curb excess calorie consumption. However, diets extremely low in fat can be often unsatisfying over time. In addition, it is important to have an adequate intake of healthy fats, especially the essential omega-3 fatty acids, and to include sufficient fat-soluble vitamins (A, D, E and K) in the regular diet. In the absence of dairy products, supplementary calcium is usually indicated to makeup the likely deficit.

Dr. Dean Ornish's Life Choice Program

What Nathan Pritikin did for patients, Dr. Dean Ornish did for professionals. He is a Clinical Professor of Medicine at the University of California (UCSF). For the past 25 years he has led a research effort, including some randomized clinical trials, which demonstrated for the first time, that the progression of even severe coronary artery disease can often be reversed by making comprehensive changes in diet and lifestyle. The changes include a very low-fat, plant-based, whole foods diet, as well as stress management techniques, moderate exercise, smoking cessation and psychosocial support. His research publications have placed him right out front in the academic community and his popular books and media appearances have made him almost a household name.

Just as with the Pritikin Diet, the change to low-fat (reduced calories) in the Ornish diet also led to observed weight loss. Who could therefore resist repackaging and remarketing this as an effective weight loss program? That's exactly what happened. Dr. Ornish's latest book, *Eat More, Weigh Less* (New York: Quill, 2001) presented a program for losing weight safely, while eating abundantly. It illustrates clearly an attempt to capitalize on this huge market. The question remains though, does the weight loss observed have any direct correlation with the specifics of this low-fat diet, other than the simple reduction in overall calories? In any case, the other cardiovascular benefits justify the calculated changes in the overall diet and lifestyle program.

The 'Ornish Diet' is almost vegetarian too, excluding all cooking oils and animal products except non-fat milk and yogurt. Moderate amounts of protein are included, mainly in the form of egg whites or vegetable protein, like that found in beans and legumes. The diet recommends avoiding chicken and fish. It excludes even high-fat plant foods like avocados, nuts and seeds. It does not limit the amount of food you can eat but advocates a kind of 'grazing' throughout the day, rather than having three big meals.

Both Pritikin and Ornish were on to something but it has become clear that low fat diets aren't always the answer. How else would one explain that 60% of the South African population is overweight, despite a comparatively low fat intake (about 22% of calories from fat) (2). In any case, many people might have difficulty sticking to such rigid diets for life. They could become tiresome very quickly because of the severe food limitations. In addition, there is some evidence that very low fat diets could result in some nutrient inadequacies. Supplementation with both minerals and vitamins, as well as essential fatty acids, would therefore be highly desirable.

And then, there is the radical view from another camp who argue against this low fat approach because it emphasizes too much carbohydrate. They insist that that is the real culprit.

છ

HIGH PROTEIN DIETS
Could Be Dangerous

In direct contrast to the low-calorie, low-fat diets of Pritikin and Ornish, for example, some controversial diets emphasizing low-carbohydrate and high-protein have become surprisingly popular over the past three decades. In the 1970's, *The Complete Scarsdale Medical Diet* and *Dr. Atkin's Diet Revolution* burst onto the diet stage with a bang. Both of these diets are based on the hypothesis that too many carbohydrates prevent the body from burning fat. They advocate that dieters should therefore fill up on protein and limit their carbohydrate-rich foods. The argument goes that excess intake of dietary carbohydrate causes the over production of insulin from the pancreas. This anabolic hormone promotes fat storage and increases appetite. That's bad news for the frustrated dieter.

High protein diets had been the mainstay for serious athletes and bodybuilders since their prized muscle mass is essentially a form of *protein* storage. But how could this become ideal for those people anxious to lose undesirable fat, especially since dense protein sources also tend to be high in fat, not to mention the feared cholesterol. The theory seemed totally contradictory to the fundamentals of good nutrition. Predictably, the professionals - doctors, nutritionists and scientists - took major issue with both Atkins and Scarsdale even though their diets gained increasing popularity and became fads in their own right. Bestselling books pushed their diet train even faster and the debate waged on.

In more recent times, Dr. Atkins has come out with his *Dr. Atkins New Diet Revolution* which presents more of the same controversial claims. To be frank, the latest offering is neither new or revolutionary. It is simply Dr. Atkins rehashing the original version of his unbalanced high-fat diet, in rather arrogant fashion, for this latest generation of quick-fix dieters trapped by their own vanity and gullibility.

Dr. Atkins says it best in the preface to his latest book. He claims that "*more than two out of every 100 adults in America has obtained a copy of this book, and more have read it. All of these readers have been forced to consider the possibility that one person may be right and the rest of the world wrong.*" That would be eminently remarkable.

The Atkins Diet

Let's briefly outline the key elements of the Atkins Diet. It consists mainly of pure protein (lean meats), pure fats (oils, butter and cream) and combinations of both proteins and fats (regular meat), with extremely small amounts of fruit and vegetables. It includes no milk, bread or starchy vegetables.

The program follows four distinct phases. First, there is a 14-day Induction phase designed to correct what is presumed to be your unbalanced metabolism. For this you are allowed to eat unlimited fat and protein, but you must restrict your carbohydrate intake to just 15-20 grams. In the second phase, Ongoing Weight Loss, you are allowed 15-40 grams of carbohydrate (from some 200 foods). As you near your target weight, you begin phase 3, Pre Maintenance, where you slowly begin to add one, two, then three weekly servings of relatively high carbohydrate foods. This gets you up to your Final Maintenance phase where you then have a mere 40-90 grams of carbohydrates per day. This is equivalent to a maximum of 360 calories which is far below the 50-60% of daily calories from carbohydrates that the vast majority of nutritionists would currently recommend for good health. That latter recommendation is for more than 250 grams(1,000 calories) of carbohydrates in a normal diet of just 2000+ calories.

This diet may have become popular because it does provide initial weight loss, probably arising mainly from water loss, appetite loss and reduced intake of calories and total food. A recent study presented at the annual meeting of the North American Associates for the Study of Obesity found that people following the Atkins diet cut their food intakes by an average of 1000 calories per day. Since 3,500 calories is equivalent to one pound of body mass, that would be more than enough to account for the dramatic weight loss that some of these dieters report.

More importantly, it indulges the dieter with the inclusion of favorite things like bacon and eggs or omelets for breakfast (no toast or juice) and unrestricted amounts of meat, fish, cheese and poultry. It seems to demand little sacrifice and that certainly has appeal for anyone in search of a quick-and-easy fix.

There are many concerns with this Atkins diet. The author is himself a trained cardiologist but one who thrives on controversy. We still have to conclude that his diet is far too high in protein and fat, and at the same time, it is far too low in carbohydrates. High proteins make excessive demands on the kidneys. High fat (triglyceride) has significant cardiovascular implications (atherosclerosis) and is associated with increased incidence of some cancers. Further, you cannot ignore the cholesterol often associated with these types of foods.

In particular, the suggestion that carbohydrate restriction compels the body to burn fat stores for energy is without much merit. This effect could produce some chemicals called ketones which are excreted in the urine. The research demonstrates however, that the daily excretion of ketones is typically equivalent to no more than 100 calories per day. That is certainly not enough to account for any amazing weight losses. But high levels of blood ketones suppress the appetite and that restricts total calorie intake. More dangerously, if ketones are allowed to build up (in a condition clinically known as ketosis), that can cause headaches, dizziness, fatigue, nausea, bad breath, and also exacerbate existing medical conditions like gout and kidney disease.

Adding to all this, the low fiber content can lead to potential constipation. Then the neglect of fruits and vegetables minimizes the valuable nutrients and phytochemicals that they contain, and which we now know can decrease the risk of cancer and heart disease. There is more. The Atkins diet is also low in calories, magnesium, potassium, vitamin C and folate. Hence, vitamin and mineral supplements should be indicated. And Dr. Atkins is pleased to provide his own brand.

The simple redeeming feature of this diet, apart from its overwhelming popularity as a fad-diet, may be the fact that high-protein foods can slow the rate of carbohydrate absorption to help maintain stable sugar levels and keep hunger at bay. Yet Dr. Atkins claims stunning success with his 25,000 overweight patients, who have been reported to take an average of 30 nutritional pills along with their daily diets. The Atkins Diet has only just become the subject of formal studies. The latest was financed by the Robert C. Atkins Foundation in New York City. Dr. Eric Westman, an internist at Duke University's diet and fitness center, studied 120 overweight volunteers in a randomized trial (3). He compared the Atkins diet against the American Heart Association's (AHA) Step 1 diet, a widely used low fat fare. With the Atkins diet, the subjects limited their carbohydrates to 20 grams a day and consumed 60 percent of their calories as fat.

The results were surprising, to say the least. After six months, those on the Atkins diet lost 31 pounds compared to 20 pounds on the AHA diet. The Atkins diet also produced better changes in cholesterol and triglyceride profiles. Two earlier preliminary studies also showed similar results. But there is a caveat - a compounding variable. It is by no means clear that these favorable changes in blood lipids can be attributed to the Atkins diet itself, since the subjects on the Atkins Diet used omega-3 oil supplements known to affect serum lipids. Those on the

AHA diet did not use these supplements. The jury must remain out on that score. A more thorough year long study, sponsored by the National Institute of Health and directed by Dr. Gary Foster of the University of Pennsylvania, will report on 300 patients.

For now, the researchers agree that much more research is necessary before this radical diet can be given broad endorsement. Possible long term health effects and the maintenance of the early weight loss must still be considered. At least, those early results will keep the Atkin's diet in the park, if not at center field. In any case, the isolated documented results with this high fat, low-carb diet do not discount the fact that many people maintain weight better on a low fat diet. Neither does it refute the fact that high consumption of fruits, vegetables and whole grains is associated with better health in hundreds of large published studies.

The Scarsdale Diet

This diet derives its name from the Medical Center where Dr. Herman Tarnover practiced medicine in Scarsdale, New York for many years. In the 1970's he developed this fad diet with some common sense added to limited clinical experience, by simply reducing caloric intake to provide fast, but from most recent accounts, temporary weight loss. *The Complete Scarsdale Medical Diet* was also introduced to the world just at the time when the obsession with physical appearance in the television age was taking off and it rode a tidal wave to popularity and success. You always knew that timing is everything. The mass market paperback proclaiming the virtues of this diet claims to be "the world's bestselling diet book ever." True or not, that's little reflection on its virtue as a truly effective weight loss program.

The Scarsdale diet promises to deliver fast results: one-pound-per-day weight loss as long as you follow the specific low-calorie intake (a daily average of 1000 calories). This includes specific fruits and vegetable portions but moderate amounts of fat from mostly lean sources of protein. It encourages also the use of artificial sweeteners and even herbal appetite suppressants to accelerate the weight loss. There is even suggestion that the combination of low carbohydrate and moderately high protein affords chemical reactions in the daily menus which somehow lead to weight loss. This strict three-meals-a-day is so low in both calories and nutrients, that one cannot survive on this diet for long periods. In fact, the plan itself only advocates two weeks on and then two weeks off, when you are allowed a few hundred more calories on the Keep Trim Program. It's no surprise then that it does not include exercise, for it could hardly fuel the normal person who walks vigorously for more than half an hour every day.

In a nutshell, this is the classic fad diet that the public has grown suspicious of. It promises to deliver what it cannot keep. There is initial success in losing weight but then one loses more than just that and cannot sustain an efficient lifestyle over time.

Surely, there must be other alternatives.

CARBOHYDRATE CONTROLS
You Don't Need

Of the three major classes of foods that provide calories in the diet, we've seen first the focus on low-fat to reduce the calorie density as in the *Pritikin Diet* and the *Dr. Dean Ornish Program*. We've then looked at the more controversial approach of focusing on reducing carbohydrates as the culprit, while allowing high-fat contributions to the diet, as in the *Atkins Diet* and the *Scarsdale Diet*. Those, in a sense, represent polar extremes. More recently, a somewhat different approach has focused not on the low-fat or high-protein (low carbohydrate) considerations, but on the intrinsic nature of carbohydrates in terms of the effect on insulin and blood sugar levels. The first diet of this type captures the guilty dieter and labels the addiction that needs to be broken. You guessed it: it's an addiction to carbohydrates.

The Carbohydrate Addict's Diet

Combine a research biologist and a psychologist who between them stand to lose 200 pounds of unwanted fat. Have them develop their own diet plan and have others join them in successful weight loss and maintenance, and you've got another diet plan to market. And that they have - with unusual success.

This couple first popularized their theory more than a decade ago in *The Carbohydrate Addict's Diet* (Dutton Books, 1991). The authors,

Dr. Richard F. Heller and Rachel F. Heller advise that you aim to control your surging insulin levels in order to lose weight. You can do this by eating two meals a day with no carbohydrates allowed. This in turn reduces your craving. Then you follow with a "reward meal" in which you are allowed a certain ratio (one third- one third- one third) with choice carbohydrates. This breaks the cycle of addiction, they claim. "Carb addicts" who previously experienced hunger, weakness, irritability, dizziness and lack of concentration after their indulgence, now avoid their usual insulin surge and the disastrous blood sugar plunge which gave rise to these effects.

The idea sounds plausible enough until the scientific research is introduced. The truth is that insulin resistance and the percentage of carbohydrates in the diet *per se* have no bearing on what is observed as weight loss success. Results show that it's the energy intake (as calories) that determines the actual weight loss and not the actual fat or carbohydrate content. Insulin resistance does not really impact on a person's ability to lose weight. It is still your net caloric intake (and to a lesser extent of course, your energy expenditure) that ultimately impacts your effective weight change. Yet the moderation exercised by avoiding high-fat and high-carbohydrate can limit overall caloric intake on this Addict's Diet for sure. That will make you lose some weight. High protein content will also reduce your appetite while the low carbohydrate can cause some initial fluid loss. So again, it may be a simple case of low calorie dieting giving the right result (in the short term), even if for the wrong reason.

The Zone Diet

Enter the Zone (Harper Collins, 1995) a dietary roadmap by biochemist Barry Sears, Ph.D. is just the latest rendition of the still popular insulin control diet. Success breeds success, so this runaway bestseller opened the floodgate for a series of four Zone Diet books and even a Zone cookbook. The Zone is appealing and even sexy, but hardly scientific.

The Zone is defined as some metabolic state in which the body works with peak efficiency, making you free from hunger, providing you with greater energy and physical performance, and giving you improved mental focus and productivity. That's the status of most professional athletes. Add in the likes of Madonna and the cast of Baywatch who are all supposed to be in the Zone, and you've got a winning prototype for millions to aspire to. Who could resist that offer? It's ideal, it's groovy, it's trendy. But is it for real?

In real terms, the Zone is really nothing more than a range of levels of insulin, which every student of diabetes has been aware of since Banting and Best first made their discovery. Every responsible diabetic does everything to monitor and control that very thing so that their levels of insulin are neither too high or too low for their own comfort and health. They know the symptoms of being outside 'the Zone'. Normal individuals can experience some of the same feelings when careless and erratic eating causes large swings in blood glucose levels. Ordinarily, the insulin response is under effective endogenous control if there is pancreatic sufficiency and adequate insulin receptors. Staying in the Zone should not be rocket science. But Sears pretends that the '*real cause of our growing epidemic of obesity is excess production of the hormone insulin. It is excess insulin that makes you fat and keeps you fat.*' That's just what some dieters would love to hear. Identify the enemy - real or imagined - and fire! And that they do.

To make the imaginative concept practical, foods are divided into blocks: protein blocks, carbohydrate blocks and fat blocks. The daily menu is then devised by combining units from different blocks to attain the magical mix for each meal or allowable snack. The plan actually turns out to allow only about 800 to 1200 calories per day which would cause almost any one to lose weight, whether these inadequate calories are derived from fat, protein or carbohydrates. This inadequacy cannot be maintained in the long run. The diet is particularly hard on dairy and wheat products (again, a trendy option), except that the valuable nutrients in these foods must be substituted of necessity.

The focus on eliminating refined grains and sugars is consistent with contemporary understanding of the glycemic response. What's that? These foods are digested too quickly and cause rapid rise in blood sugar levels. As such, they are said to have a high *glycemic index* and therefore stimulate high insulin secretion. This leads to a drain of blood glucose that zaps your energy and much more. Insulin drives glucose into storage (as fat) and inhibits the conversion of existing body fat back into glucose. It is therefore clearly crucial to maintain relatively low insulin levels for effective weight loss and that means avoiding foods with a high glycemic index. More on that later.

The focus on the role of insulin is welcome in a fast food society where there is so much appeal to the sweet tooth and irresponsible indulgence. Although controlling insulin inside the Zone, whatever that really means, may have other connotations, it does not contain the final solution to weight loss by any means.

A more pragmatic and defensible plan is presented in *The Glycemic Index Diet* (Random House, 2002) by Rick Gallop who formalized this approach after the original research of Professor David Jenkins at my Alma Mater, the University of Toronto. Using the glycemic index (GI) for foods that Jenkins published in 1980, Gallop devised a diet plan to overcome what he calls '*the major problems of dieting, namely complexity and hunger.*' He lists foods in one of three color-coded categories based on their glycemic index: foods to avoid, foods to eat occasionally and foods to eat as much as you want. There is much to commend in this sensible approach to weight management, but it is not a comprehensive solution.

Sugar Busters (Ballatine Books, 2nd Edition, 1998) is yet another popular high-protein, low-carbohydrate diet where the emphasis is on the toxicity of sugar. That simple claim is that sugar makes you fat. That's the enemy, along with all refined carbohydrates. Popular success of this trendy title has spawned a shopper's guide, cookbooks and even a special version for kids.

This diet was developed by three physicians and the CEO of a Fortune 500 company, which suggests where it may be coming from and where it's wanting to go. It's another fad diet in search of a wave to carry it to the shore of financial success. Sugar is a convenient target and fighting it appeals to common sense, especially to all those struggling with their weight, yet suffering from the guilt of sweet indulgence with irresistible desserts and with fast, convenience and junk foods that haunt their daily existence. It sounds appealing, yes, but hardly original for it's nothing more than a new marketable spin on the same insulin story.

It is difficult to find what's new or what's more than hype in this protocol. Perhaps, it's the fact that it allows more carbohydrate than say, The Atkins Diet, but insists on the complex variety like whole grains, fruits and vegetables. As such, it is fairly well-balanced and puts up a warning flag for all those empty calories in foods loaded with simple sugars and in refined carbohydrates. That's a large portion of the typical American diet and does contribute to the obesity epidemic for sure.

However, it's the fundamental premise that is in question. They may have the theory all backwards: it's more likely that obesity will cause insulin resistance, rather than insulin resistance induced by dietary habit will cause obesity.

Here's the bottom line. The weight loss observed on these low carbohydrate sugar-free diets may reflect more on the overall limits to caloric intake than on anything else. Cutting back on simple sugars makes intuitive sense, but they focus on carbohydrate controls you don't really need. Insulin, we will see in the next chapter, cannot be made a scapegoat for your weight problem.

COMBO PLANS
That Make No Sense

We've seen different approaches to dieting by zeroing in on the three major classes of foods that provide calories in the diet. They all have their limitations but sooner or later, as you would expect, others would conceive entirely different strategies. Some have focused on what we now classify today as food combining.

Back in the 1930's, this popular concept originated with an early diet book by one William Hay, who daringly advocated that starch should not be consumed at the same time with proteins, and fruits should not be eaten with either of these.

But this hypothesis we now clearly understand, holds no water at all. Needless to say, digestion is a well orchestrated process, controlled by specific enzymes secreted at different times in different parts of the digestive tract. The whole process is designed to cope with very acidic juices from the stomach and then the alkaline secretions from the pancreas and small intestine, all acting in concert. To help facilitate this, foods rich in carbohydrates are first to leave the stomach, while fats and proteins slow down the dumping from the stomach.

Nevertheless, this simplistic idea of combining foods for advantage, to lose weight, has given rise more recently to a number of popular fad diets. For example, Judy Mazel was an aspiring actress but became more of a self-styled nutrition guru to the stars. This gave her leverage to launch her first bestseller *The Beverly Hills Diet* (Reprint edition, Buccaneer Books,1981). It was a small but incredibly popular book that laid out a fairly strict diet plan for quick and easy weight loss.

The Beverly Hills Diet was an unusual innovation, starting off with nothing but fruits for the first ten days. There was lots of fruit for sure. You could eat a half pound of prunes at one sitting or five pounds of grapes in a single day, for example. Anybody would lose weight initially on that menu. Then came the addition of bread and butter leading up to a meal with complete protein only near the end of week three.

Needless to say, the title of this diet alone made it appealing. You could identify with the stars and share in the lives of the rich and famous. If this diet was good enough for them, then clearly, it would be good for you too. Add the simplicity, the structure, the guaranteed early weight loss and even the allowance of a little fatty dessert treat and voilà, a perfect fad diet. Lots of variety came later in the plan but then came back the weight too. Like a true fad diet, it had no sustainability and in the long run, could even prove unhealthy.

The New Beverly Hills Diet is a variant on the same old incoherent theme. It broadens the food choices somewhat in a new 35-day program but it remains essentially fruit and more fruit, so its nutritional shortcomings are still evident. Ms. Mazel destroys any residual credibility by her disregard for the important role of exercise and physical activity which hardly fits into her major indefensible premise.

Other variants on this diet were hardly any better. Most still liked the idea of nothing but fruits in the morning. Some even went further than that and like *The Hollywood Diet* dating back to the 1930's, emphasized little else on the menu but grapefruits, which they falsely claimed had some special enzyme that had the capacity to burn-away fat. In fact, proponents of this fruit-based, food-combining plan, made even more exaggerated claims that 'papaya softens body fat, pineapple burns it off and watermelon flushes it out of the body.' Sounds ideal, doesn't it? Unreal, too.

But could there be something here? Should this lead us to do some lateral thinking, thinking outside the box, if you like? Could enzymes actually have a critical role? Are we perusing the right superstar players - those enzymes - but assuming the wrong role for them?

That's intriguing. We'll come back to this in Part II of this book when we address **The Enzyme Diet™** and its unique focus. What we do know for certain is that people lost weight on these diets but that was essentially from what could almost be called, mere 'starvation.' The combining or non-combining of different food classes had little or nothing to do with the apparent weight loss. All such semi-starvation diets will cause weight loss but they are too unhealthy to be followed seriously for any length of time.

DIET PROGRAMS
That Can Control You

Speaking of following diets for a long time, dieting itself, one must admit, is a personal challenge. It should not be compared with smoking cessation or alcohol withdrawal, but it is still a form of behavior modification that does not come easily for everyone. Historically, dieters have often faced the challenges of a bruised self-image, of boring self-discipline and frequently, inadequate social adjustment. This combined reality created the need for group support and/or personal counseling, at least for those who obviously needed some kind of help, as they struggled to cope with their weight management. Some dieters seem to have found the answer there. What they could not do by themselves, they managed to achieve with support from others and sometimes even with external control.

Weight Watchers
This is the mother of all weight loss programs. Since 1963 more than 23 million people have participated in these small groups in their efforts to lose a few or many unwanted pounds. Each local group is led by a successful Weight Watchers graduate who is later trained with leadership skills and certified by the program. Weekly meetings are opportunities to weigh-in, to discuss the challenges that all dieters face, to exchange coping strategies, to gain moral support and regain acceptance, and to trade ideas for meal planning and menu alternatives.

The bottom-line is still counting calories. A point system for some 12,000 foods, based on calories, fat and fiber, allows each participant to be somewhat flexible while they consume a specific number of points each day, based on one's weight and defined goals. There is no encouragement for crash dieting. Rather, the program calls for three steps. The goal in Step One is simply to lose that first 10% of weight. Step Two is designed to help you achieve your target weight and naturally, Step Three is designed for maintenance - often the biggest challenge. You can eat virtually anything as long as you keep within your allotted points for each day. If you misbehave or indulge, you can compensate with fewer points the next day. You even get to keep a journal or diary that helps make you accountable, even to yourself.

Weight watchers is careful to stress the value of physical activity and exercise as a valuable part of their program. After all, if counting calories is the focus - the *raison d'etre* - the importance of caloric intake must be balanced by the obvious expenditure of those calories. Only the difference in the *calorie balance equation* determines the net effect, resulting in the desired weight loss. Whether you diet for yourself, by yourself or in the context of an accountable group, the mathematics is still the same.

The Weight Watcher's program works well for some people. *Lifetime members* report that after completing the maintenance phase of the program, they have kept off an average of 84% of their weight loss. That's not bad at all. But maybe that's why they are the select lifetime members. About half of these even report that they were at the 100% mark after two years. *Hat's off* to them! But what of the millions who have gone through the program and just plain given up in frustration? They got tired of counting calories, bored by weekly meetings, disillusioned by slow results and who knows what else. The net result was that they packed it in.

Weight Watchers continues to be popular and recently got a boost from the Duchess of York who wrote "*Dieting with the Duchess*" (by Sarah Ferguson and Sarah Mountbatten-Win York, Fireside Publishers, 2000) to further popularize their calorie-counting plan. Needless to say, association with royalty does nothing for your struggle to lose weight and keep it off, but as Marshall Macluhan would say, '*the medium becomes the message'* in a royal *figure* (pun intended).

Jenny Craig

Here's a variant on the flexible Weight Watchers program that advocates structure and discipline. It's a program that was developed by registered dieticians and psychologists with some input from medical doctors. Leave it to professional beavers. They've got the answers, they'll take control. They even provide their own brand of prepackaged foods, complemented with some additional supermarket foods and Jenny Craig's "weight loss supplements."

Clients attend weekly lifestyle classes and one-on-one counseling sessions. They are taught how to tailor their individual diet regimes to get somewhere between 1000 and 2600 calories per day, depending on their gender and current weight. Imagine someone else designing your eating menu and even providing your food. They do emphasize increased physical activity, changing some poor ingrained eating habits and learning how to balance meals and food choices. But after losing half of one's goal weight, clients are given an option to make the transition to regular foods. That's where the rubber meets the road. It's difficult no matter what, to get enough real-life preparation on how to choose one's own menu to get adequate nutrition from commercial low calorie foods. This is even more true after using a crutch, where someone else does it for you. There is no published research data on the success rates for Jenny Craig members but obviously, the program has made inroads into the market place. Advertising plays a significant role, especially after the brief run of ads which featured the household name and figure of one Monica Lewinsky. It's intriguing to wonder if the consuming public made the comparison to that other spokesperson, Sarah Ferguson, Duchess of York. Or could they not get past the higher notoriety?

POTPOURRI PLANS
Can Be Way Off

There is no limit to the creative imagination. A lucrative opportunity awaits any novel idea that promises to bring relief to those desperate to find a panacea for their weight challenge. So a host of would be diet gurus have emerged over the years, promoting hundreds of new approaches or new spins on old ideas. In recent years a few of these have become popular and any review of contemporary diets would be incomplete without at least a mention of a few of them.

Eat Right 4 Your Type

Here's a good example of a theory that makes no biological sense. A second generation Doctor of Naturopathic Medicine, Peter D'Adamo, put forward the ridiculous notion that a person's blood type determines his or her susceptibility to illness. *Eat Right 4 Your Type* (G.P. Putman's Sons, 1996) was co-authored with Catherine Whitney and promoted as the individualized diet solution to staying healthy, living longer and achieving your ideal weight. Initial success has led to five other follow-up books including an encyclopedia and two cookbooks. Your blood type, they surmise, represents an important part of your biological heritage. It reflects your ancestral roots and even the original dietary habits of your people.

The immediate question for any informed person would be: which of the different blood group systems is indicative. The ABO system, although perhaps the most significant clinically, for reasons of compatibility and blood transfusion, is only one of several distinguishing characteristics of human cells. The ABO system refers to the presence or absence of some specific, genetically-determined molecular structures (antigens) on the membranes of red blood cells in particular. But there are other systems of more importance for other responses. Take for example, the so-called Rh system. This affects the compatibility of mother's blood, which may or may not have an Rh marker, with that of the newborn baby who also possibly carries an Rh marker from the father. This can cause the possible incompatibility with subsequent children. That could lead to serious illness and even death. What could be more important?

How on earth could a given ABO blood type dictate the types of food to be tolerated by an individual or even worse, the potential healing powers of each body? This idea is as elusive as it is opportunistic. And why the red blood cells? Why not the white blood cells which we know are the critical defenders of the immune system? Why not cells of the brain or perhaps the endocrine system, which have such dominant systemic control?

But weight loss is only one of the supposed benefits. Imagine increased resistance to infection, reduced risk of cancer, cardiovascular disease, diabetes, liver failure and even anti-aging. All this, D'Adamo claims, and not a shred of evidence is offered except the years of unpublished research that he and his father carried out in this field. Whatever became of Science! Yet these books fly off store shelves and a growing number of gullible disciples follow in the wake. Imagine!

The Origin Diet

Speaking of roots, author Elizabeth Somer would have us take a long leap backwards and revert to the kind of diet that our ancestors consumed in the Stone Age. In the good old days, humans lived close to nature and ate lots of wild game and the fruit of the earth - plants, vegetables and fruits. What a bargain that was! There was lots of fiber to chew on and all the vitamins, minerals and phytonutrients that abound in nature. At the same time, there was adequate carbohydrate and protein, without the high fat content we know today. Obviously, there were no empty calories, so overall, it was like the best of all worlds back then. This is consistent with all that dogma coming from dieticians and nutritionists today. There's really nothing new here. But the claim is that if we could rediscover the diet of our early ancestors, the benefits could go far beyond just weight loss. The principles would even suggest that you could reduce your risk of so many diseases associated with poor nutrition even in affluent societies. Take for example, heart disease, cancer, osteoporosis, hypertension, diabetes, and the list goes on.

The big challenge here would still be to find the sources of such really low fat meats and the abundant whole grains, fresh fruit and vegetables. In our culture, the abundance of fast, convenience and processed foods and the sheer pace of life itself, all mitigate against this primitive nutritional package. Who can avoid the appeal of slick advertising, the marketing to satisfy sensual delight, the convenience of processing and packaging, or the availability of instant meals and snacks? No amount of 'hunter-gatherer' snacks or Stone Age Zinger Smoothies, could ever compete with today's fare. In essence, whatever appeal this diet may have on University Avenue it will not show up on Main Street.

Soup Diets

If you're otherwise well and just dreaming of knocking off a few pounds, here's as simple a diet solution as you could wish. It may date back originally two or three decades to an original version which called for cabbage soup, cabbage soup and more cabbage soup - plain and simple. In those days, you could add cranberry juice, some select fruits and vegetables and for a single day in the 7-day plan, you could even indulge with one serving of beef or chicken. This was a short, crash program of low calories and low fat which guaranteed the loss of at least a few pounds - maybe ten to fifteen or so.

Other versions of this soup-diet plan calls for unlimited amounts of soup and then one or more specified foods for each of seven days. Soup can be filling and serve as an effective appetite suppressant. But it can also cause gas, nausea and even light-headedness after just a few days on such a low calorie protocol. It's a fad diet that will probably yield short term weight loss but after a week or two, the questions remain: What's next? Where to from here? There must be a better alternative.

The Enzyme Diet™ Solution will show you how to lose weight and keep it off safely, effectively and conveniently. But there are other weight loss approaches that still need to be briefly reviewed here before we get into the crux of the problem.

☙

QUICK FIX DIET PILLS
Will Make You Sick

Too many people with a weight problem turn in desperation for a quick fix. They look for some magic pill that they hope could deliver what any number of diets that they may have tried have all failed to do. In our drug culture, where doctors can prescribe a therapeutic solution for almost any symptom or complaint, the public is often deluded into thinking that pills can solve them all. Add to that the endless claims of alternative practitioners with their herbal remedies, and the frustrated dieter now has a wide field to choose from.

Most diet pills fall into one of four broad classes: appetite suppressants, stimulants, fat-blockers and diuretics. Let's take a brief look at each of these. We'll soon see their harmful effects.

Appetite Suppressants
The star of this show has been commonly known as the combi-

nation drug **fen-phen**. This is the once popular drug that hit the weight loss industry with a bang in the last decade. It is a classic story of the rise and fall of incomplete or inadequate therapeutic science.

Fen-phen is the convenient abbreviation for the drug which actually contains low doses of either **fen**fluramine (Pondimin™) or dexfenfluramine (Redux™) in combination with **phen**termine (a drug which acts like an amphetamine). The action of fen-phen is essentially to alter the levels of the neurotransmitter serotonin, in the brain. This in turn, effectively blocks the impulses that would normally tell you that you're hungry. Therefore, if you took fen-phen, your appetite would be suppressed - you would consume less food (calories) and you would lose weight. That sounds very logical and simple, but it isn't.

Many years ago, both phentermine and fenfluramine had been approved by the FDA for use, on prescription, as appetite suppressants. In 1984, some research was published that suggested one could also achieve effective weight loss by using both in combination, and with fewer side effects than when the drugs were used separately. With the huge market potential, the industry pushed the development of fen-phen and by 1992, one study with 120 obese patients demonstrated an average loss of 30 pounds.

Fenfluramine gave rise to new and improved dexfenfluramine in 1995, and when that combination with phentermine hit the market with FDA approval, the weight loss industry adopted this new 'panacea' with abandon. Here, at last, was the 'magic pill' - the weight loss 'miracle-drug' - that even physicians and commercial weight loss centers adopted as the safe and effective solution for their overweight patients. Just imagine that in 1996, the first year of its mass marketing, physicians wrote more than 17 million prescriptions for about 6 million dieters. Some of these patients were truly obese and had a lot to lose, but some were on a frantic search for a method to lose a mere 5, 10 or 15 pounds. Unfortunately, they all potentially lost much more than weight.

By the summer of just the following year, 1997, the euphoria turned to sadness and shame. In July, some astute researchers at the Mayo Clinic and Foundation reported 24 cases (one third of the total) of rare valvular heart disease in women who had used the fen-phen combination. The light came on, and soon another 75 additional reports were received at the FDA. Other reports came in of similar observations in patients using fenfluramine or dexfenfluramine separately. As expected, the FDA recognized the need for prompt action and asked the manufacturers to voluntarily withdraw all these drugs off the market for the treatment of obesity. The drug companies had no choice and soon fen-phen would become a thing of the past.

That's the kind of history, one would prefer not to repeat, but as someone else has rightly said, if we wish not to repeat history we must make certain to learn from its lessons.

What are some of those lessons? Be slow to resort to therapeutics when lifestyle issues are paramount. Avoid any rush to drug approval and introduction, no matter how huge the market potential. Patients matter infinitely more than profits. When assessing risk, always err on the side of caution and when assessing benefit, separate health from everything else. Don't always follow the crowd. Too often the masses take the easy route - the path of least resistance. Even when professionals concur, there is no guarantee of safety in the long run. Those are just a few obvious conclusions to get you started. What else might you learn from this?

Valvular heart disease was actually only one of the major side effects from fen-phen. Add to this serious possibility, the prospects of primary pulmonary hypertension and neuropsychological damage to the brain. To put it simply, fen-phen was bad news! To try to decrease one's appetite with drugs is no real solution to anyone's weight problem.

Apparently, phentermine itself is still available on prescription but it should only be used, if at all, in conjunction with an overall diet plan for effective weight management. These pills should never be given to children. It is contraindicated in several medical conditions and doctors should warn their patients of what side effects to expect including sleeplessness, irritability, stomach upset or constipation.

Stimulants

Among the stimulant drugs used for weight loss, two are widely used. The first is *ephedrine* which is also an appetite suppressant. More importantly though, it stimulates the central nervous system just like the amphetamines. It revs up the system just like '*speed*'. It therefore affects the brain and cardiovascular system too. The body's metabolism artificially increases and burns up more calories by a process known as thermogenesis. In addition to the ephedrine, the second drug *caffeine* is usually included in these weight loss stimulant drugs. The effect of the ephedrine is thereby enhanced.

Ephedrine is popular among herbal practitioners as the active ingredient in extracts of *Chinese Ephedrine* or *Ma Huang* (one type of ephedra). It has been used in Chinese Medicine for a variety of ailments but it acts physiologically on many different systems which makes its side effects quite common. It is commonly used three times a day in the form of a tea, a tincture or an extract.

Caffeine is used by the alternative practitioners in the form of a Brazilian cocoa known usually as *guarana*. Guarana is used not only for weight loss, but also to enhance athletic performance and reduce fatigue. It has properties which endear it to folk medicine claims as a tonic, aphrodisiac, diuretic and astringent, as well as a remedy for common ailments. The seed which is commonly used contains 2.5-7 percent pure caffeine, compared to 1-2 percent in regular coffee. For weight loss purposes, 1-2 capsules or tablets of guarana containing 200-800 mg of the extract is typically used before breakfast and lunch.

Ephedrine and caffeine can be used separately or in combination, but the effect is similar and synergistic. These stimulants can be quite invigorating but the side effects alone mitigate against them.

Yet ephedra is widely sold across the United States. The government continues to delay limiting its use until it has conclusive results from ongoing studies of its safety. You could find it in some pharmacies, groceries, health food stores, fitness clubs, gas stations, and of course on the Internet and even on TV infomercials. Some good estimates put its consumption as high as 3 billion doses per year. The American Herbal Products Association reported that sales of ephedra approached $1 billion in 1999. Unbelievable!

Products containing ephedra account for less than one percent of the total herbal supplement sales in the US. However, these products were responsible for 62 percent of all herbal-related reports made to poison control centers nationwide in 2002. Researchers calculated that the use of ephedra poses a risk 200 times greater than the risks posed by all other herbal supplements combined. It is clearly unsafe for routine and unsupervised use.

Ephedra is still a banned substance for athletes in the NFL, NCAA and the Olympics. In Canada, the Consumer Protection Branch of Health Canada (the Canadian equivalent of the FDA) launched a voluntary recall of certain ephedra products, based on at least sixty reports of adverse events including a likely death.

Even if you are lucky enough to never experience any of these serious side effects, there are consequences of long-term use of stimulants. Most people (more than 95%) who use thermogenic products for weight loss will gain the weight back plus some, after discontinuing use of the product. So you put yourself at risk for what? A few days or weeks of being 'wired'? That's no solution at all.

Fat Blockers

In a world of advertised "low-fat" and "non-fat" foods, it's no wonder fat is thought of as the "bad buy". Unfortunately, up until recently, there was a media and therefore cultural obsession with being lean and almost too thin. When coupled with the misconceptions about fat per se and its role in health, this has led to a fat-free version of nearly all foods, from potato chips to brownies. This "low-fat" frenzy has also spawned the development of synthetic products such as fat blockers and fat substitutes.

An example of a fat blocker is the drug Orlistat (Xenical®) which acts by blocking the action of the fat digestive enzymes (lipases) in the stomach and small intestine. The drug itself is not absorbed and is administered typically as a capsule three times a day with main meals. At this dosage, fat absorption is inhibited by approximately 30%. There are reports that use of Xenical involves risks of hypertension, high cholesterol, heart disease and diabetes. It should not be used by people who suffer from malabsorption syndrome or have reduced bile flow.

As you might expect, there is a natural alternative already on the market. It is a product known as *chitosan* which is a dietary fiber-like substance made from chitin. Chitin itself forms the hard shells of crabs, lobsters and other shell fish. It binds to fat and other fat-soluble substances. The clinical effects of chitosan on cholesterol and triglycerides in the blood remain unclear, with conflicting research data. However, while it is theorized that chitosan is a fat blocker and might help aid in weight reduction, clinical trials with chitosan show no effect on weight loss [4].

Many people see the commercials for these fat blockers and fat substitutes and think that they are just what they need to help them lose weight. Unfortunately, blocking fats and eating synthetic fat substitutes come with their share of problems too, including digestive problems and diarrhea.

A bigger problem lies in the fact that these fat blockers or fat substitutes prevent the body from absorbing the fat we do eat. Despite what many diets and commercials promote, the truth is that not all fat is bad. We need some fat. The 'good fats' are called essential fats or essential fatty acids (EFAs). These good fats cannot be made by your body and must be included in your diet. Essential fatty acids, like protein and carbohydrates, are absolutely essential nutrients. Without them, you might experience many of the following symptoms of EFA deficiency: brittle nails or hair, bleeding gums, poor circulation (cold hands and feet), dry skin, oily or dry hair, excessive hair loss, candidiasis, excessive thirst and lowered resistance to infections and disease.

The fact is that fat itself is essential for health. Along with being the most concentrated food energy source available, fat provides cushioning for vital organs, promotes healthy skin and hair, regulates cholesterol metabolism, affects hormone production and aids in the transport and absorption of fat-soluble vitamins. Whether you avoid fat or block it, the fat is unavailable for use in the body, meaning you lose out on the benefits this fat provides.

Fat substitutes and fat blockers prevent the absorption of essential fat-soluble vitamins A, D, E and K. This means you miss out on all the health benefits which include keeping the immune system healthy and reducing the risk of prostate cancer, lung cancer, heart disease and macular degeneration (deteriorating eyesight).

A third problem is that fat substitutes and fat blockers can bind or trap some minerals, thus preventing their absorption. This means you get less of the important minerals like calcium, magnesium, and iron into your body and to the cells that need them. When cells don't get the nutrients they need, they 'starve' and your metabolism slows. In other words, using fat blockers or fat substitutes can sabotage your metabolism, your weight loss efforts and your health.

Diuretics

It is a well known observation that a major contributor to the excess weight of each concerned individual is the net retention of excess fluid (water). Water is regulated in the body through several mechanisms including fluid intake, kidney excretion, fecal output, evaporation from the skin and water vapor in exhaled air and speech. This balance is intricately controlled but sometimes, by the failure of different physiological controls, excess water retention can and often does become a problem. Most people who go on a diet, find that they experience a fairly rapid initial loss, essentially due to the loss of excess water from the tissues.

This process is affected every day by doctors with the use of different kinds of drugs known as diuretics. They are clinically chosen for their varied potency and other characteristics. The use of diuretics can have significant medical side effects and potential complications and should only be administered under the supervision of a medical doctor. There is an appropriate role for this type of intervention in the management of obesity but since it is reserved for professional application, it need not be discussed any further here. However, it must always be stressed that even when diuretics are prescribed as part of a weight management plan, that plan must always be comprehensive to address all the lifestyle factors of nutrition, supplementation and exercise, in particular.

So far in this chapter, we have selectively reviewed for you a wide variety of popular diet products and programs on the market in America today. We presumptuously set out to find why your last weight loss diet probably failed - just as it has for the remaining 95% of dieters just like you. We found that low fat diets are not the whole story and aren't always the answer. High protein diets are extremely popular today but can be dangerous. Attempts to manipulate insulin are not grounded in science and focus on carbohydrate controls you don't need. Various combination plans do no justice to your highly specialized digestive enzymes. Each of these diets may cause you to lose weight initially, but often for the wrong reason and for the short term only. Many dieters turn in desperation for counseling and support. Group programs still focus on calories and tend to usurp your personal control of your weight loss program. After all, it's your problem and you must find your personal life-long solution. You need something simple and effective. Diet pills are not magic pills and pose far more problems than they solve. They could make you sick, so the remedy remains elusive.

However, there is one approach that we are yet to discuss in this dieting panorama. *Meal Replacements* **represent a proven, effective strategy that could very well be the way for you to go.**

ç

A MEAL REPLACEMENT
Could Be The Solution!

We have looked at the different classes of foods that contribute the calories that lead to the storage of excess as body fat. We also discussed several strategies that have allowed different authors to devise diets that lead to weight loss. Essentially, it seems that most if not all these diets have but one thing in common. Reduce caloric intake and Bingo! ... you see weight loss results. But up to now, we have considered only different permutations and combinations of naturally-occurring foods in a standard menu format. However, for many decades, different promoters have devised special concoctions that can best be described as Meal Replacements **either** as a nutritional boost like a fast, instant meal, or as a meal substitute designed to deliver the nutritional benefits of a normal meal but without the unwanted calories. As we shall see, this latter strategy is ideally suited for a weight loss diet program.

The idea is not new. A doctor in Chicago was pushing his own formula "*Dr. Stoll's Diet-Aid, the Natural Reducing Food*" before the last world war. He made a blend of milk chocolate, starch, whole wheat and bran, and promoted a formula of "one teaspoon in a cup of water" in place of breakfast and then of lunch. That was clearly a poor start to what has now become a huge industry that pervades homes, supermarkets, pharmacies, hospitals and many other institutions. Liquid formulas, powders, shakes, bars, biscuits and the like have become standard meal replacements and food snacks.

The liquid diets were extremely popular back in the 1970's, but then they got a bad rap with the introduction of some poorly devised liquid protein diets which had some adverse and even fatal consequences. However, in more recent time, a new generation of nutritionally-balanced formulas have been introduced to the market and have combined the appeal of convenience and good balanced nutrition, with or without calories, depending on intended use.

Several studies have shown that when dieters were given meal replacements as part of a reduced calorie food plan, they lost more weight than those prescribed the same number of calories with no meal replacements. A recent review of data from 29 studies of overweight and obese people who participated in weight loss programs in the US, led the authors to the conclusion **that meal replacements make it easier for people to follow a restricted energy (very low calorie) regimen** (5). They found that those who lost more weight (about 44 pounds) were more likely to maintain their weight loss over time than those who lost less than 22 pounds. They attributed this to the bigger incentive for the first group to keep the weight off, than persons who lose 15-20 pounds but are still obese. People who lose more weight have more time and energy invested in their weight success and may have learned more in the process. Individuals who exercised the most were also more likely to keep weight off than those who did little exercise. No surprise there.

Long-term follow up is obviously important. The limited data points in a favorable direction for meal replacements. Long term follow up of those who have lost weight show that those using meal replacements have greater success at keeping it off. In fact, a one year follow up of weight loss in two comparable groups showed that the group using meal replacements maintained their weight loss, while the group that did not use meal replacements gained back almost all the weight that had been previously lost. A different five year follow up study yielded similar results.

David Heber, M.D. Ph.D., the Director of the UCLA Center for Human Nutrition offered *The Resolution Diet* (Avery, 1999) as a more authoritative guide to losing weight and keeping it off and clearly made a case for the wise and practical use of meal replacements in a comprehensive lifestyle strategy. He reported that published studies from the UCLA group with hundreds of participants at six different sites across the United States, reveal consistent weight loss and excellent compliance with meal replacements (6). After two years, both men and women maintained an average weight loss of about 14 pounds. Dr. Heber made further reference to several other studies which justify his claim to the effectiveness of the meal replacement method. It guarantees the best of nutrition without the burdensome task of counting daily calories and the inconvenience of structuring each meal on one's menu. It also avoids the hunger pangs, weakness and fatigue that are associated with so many extreme low-calorie 'starvation' diets.

Dr. Heber cited one study in Germany that compared the use of two meal replacements per day with simply trying to count calories in diets of 1200 to 1500 calories per day (7). The group using meal replacements lost an average of over 15 pounds, while those who simply cut back on their intake lost only 3 pounds on average after twelve weeks. Over the following two years, the meal replacement group lost an average of an additional 6.6 pounds, or an effective total of more than 20 pounds, using just one meal replacement as maintenance.

Here's an unusual community study reported by Dr. Heber. In the town of Pound, Wisconsin (an ironic twist!), the residents were given free coupons for a meal replacement to substitute for an average of one meal per day, over a five year period (1992 - 1997). During that time, while the nation as a whole was otherwise putting weight on, the participants lost and kept off an average of 9 to 12 pounds. Here's the joke. The mayor of Pound lost 42 pounds himself on the program and harmlessly suggested re-naming the town to Ounce, Wisconsin. That could have made headline news.

Media icon Oprah Winfrey certainly made news when she underwent her own makeover in the late 1980's. She used essentially a meal replacement diet to transform into a new model in tight jeans. Her world of fans applauded, but only for a while. The weight later came back, much to the disappointment of the many fans who had taken to copying all kinds of diet plans offering strawberry, chocolate and vanilla shakes. Listen to Oprah tell her story in her own words:

> *"I've been struggling with my weight since I was 22 ...*
> *I've lost and gained too many times to count. I've used*
> *food to relieve stress, for comfort, and to momentarily*
> *stand in for joy ... In 1988 the nation watched while I*
> *starved myself (using Optifast® - a meal replacement)*
> *for four months so I could fit into a pair of jeans. I got*
> *down to 145 pounds - and stayed there for one day*
> *before the regaining began. I reached my highest weight*
> *in 1992, wobbling around at 237 pounds"* (8)

This was proof-positive that some meal replacements are not in themselves the necessary answer. Most liquid diets are too low in calories (often 500 to 800 calories per day) for the typical person to follow over the long-term. They must be incorporated into a more thorough and complete strategy that provides all the essentials of nutrition including bulk fiber and of course, added to satisfying complementary meals and a proper exercise program.

Perhaps we should update the Oprah saga. She took control again in 1992 and with her new trainer Bob Greene, lost the weight again. She even ran a marathon. Four years later, with more emotional stress and career pressure, she emotionally ate her way back to around 200 pounds. Yo-yo again. She then began to have cardiovascular symptoms and that did it. Now driven of necessity, she undertook a more complete program including both cardiovascular and strength training. Today she is 33 pounds lighter and counting, while watching her dietary habits closely (8). Oprah remains just one (albeit illustrious) example of the typical success and failure of dieting and weight loss.

Today, there are a number of popular meal replacements on the market. They range in quality and effectiveness but fall into two general categories. First, there are those which provide the very low calorie, semi-fasting compositions which are more appropriate for the more obese individuals who desire or need more rapid weight loss for one reason or another. That application should only be used under medical supervision. For the more usual dieter, the other category of meal replacements is generally without much risk when used to substitute for one or two meals, and complemented with real food - low in fat, rich in nutrients and controlled for calories. That's the best of all worlds.

Not quite. It can get even better. In Part II of this book you'll discover why **The Enzyme Diet™** employs all those great advantages of the meal replacement strategy described above, but also incorporates some often neglected but important principles of nutrition and an innovative nutrient delivery system. These give it most distinct advantages for effective and healthy weight loss, and a winning difference in today's crowded marketplace. **The Enzyme Diet™ Solution** is a comprehensive program of sensible dieting, combined with moderate exercise and emotional control. That's the way to go.

Before we get there, we must go a little deeper to find out how you got a weight problem in the first place! What exactly is the crux of the problem? Why do so many dieters quit after they experience the frustration of yo-yo dieting? Why is the answer so elusive?

It's a real challenge.

Chapter 3

THE REAL CHALLENGE
Your Weight Problem - Does It Still Exist?

You now understand that there is an overweight problem in America. Chances are that since you're reading this, either you are, or someone close to you is, a part of that very problem. In the first Chapter, we emphasized that the problem is not the weight itself because apart from the fashion industry and the media, who else would care. The critical issue is not weight, but health. The health consequences of overweight and obesity are serious. It is indeed a silent epidemic and a growing one.

But all the attempts to manage weight have almost consistently led to failure and frustration. Chapter 2 was a short critical review of some limited examples of the more popular fad diets and diet pills that continue to be used by millions of people across this nation. Some are anxious to shed a few extra pounds just to improve their self-image and to conform to popular media stereotypes. Others are challenged by their increased risks for many diseases and are being urged by health care professionals, of necessity, to lose significant amounts of weight to improve their prognosis and longevity. In either case, almost half the population is likely to try something, sometime in this calendar year, to effectively reduce the amount of excess baggage they're hauling around. But most of these 'eager beavers' who set about to lose the few extra inches or the bulging bellies will soon give up with disappointment and at times, despair. Have you ever been one of those? Let's examine the ten most significant reasons why so many fail to realize their goals.

Why Dieters Quit

Reason #1.   Hunger Pangs

I'm sure you have friends who have reported to you their all-too-familiar experience. They were anxious to lose weight so they started on this fantastic diet they heard about, but soon they felt they were starving. The urge to eat led to a surge of uncontrollable passion and they went back on a splurge. They tried to contain their hunger pangs until the rising crescendo catapulted them to their favorite restaurant and that triggered everything. Or they happened to be in the refrigerator or at the supermarket and they could no longer restrain themselves. Their cells cried out for food. It was a case of '*feed us or we'll die* ' - a natural instinct, after all.

Very low calorie diets often tend to provide inadequate nutrition. That's bad news. When cells don't get an adequate supply of their essential nutrients, they get mad, they scream for help and the appetite soars. No amount of counting calories will compensate for the need of nutrients and energy to silence the cellular storm. You cannot survive on an inadequate starvation diet ... no matter what!

In contrast, **The Enzyme Diet**™ will keep you satisfied and full of energy while you lose weight.

Reason #2.   Plain Boredom

Food is fun. The variety of food is exciting. The taste of food could be pure ecstasy. Nature abounds in diversity and we are programmed to respond to all the many varieties of taste, color, aroma, mouth-feel and more...Yes, we actually use all our five senses since we can even delight in the fifth sense of sound from a kettle singing, a stew simmering or a steak sizzling. In the course of a given day, our lives are enriched by the multitude of little blessings that constitute the kaleidoscope of experience. Our experience with food is an integral part of that reality.

So, if you are confined or constrained by a very limited diet menu, you will soon become bored by the monotonous repetition of the same daily fare. Many a diet can be low in calories, low in nutrients and also low in appeal. That could be really upsetting. Imagine, you are teased by all the appealing triggers. These could range from the fanciest delicacies and appetizers to the sweetest desserts, but you are obliged to restrain yourself to the *same ol', same ol'*.   It's just like being in a culinary prison or some other institutional kitchen, where sometimes you don't even want to see or smell the *same ol' food*. You can feel at times like a cat with her chow or a dog with his kibble. That can kill the best of all dieting intentions. You must have variety. Sooner or later, grapefruit will be just grapefruit, cabbage soup will be cabbage soup and any other single item menu will become just that. Boring!

You will find a number of delicious recipes for **The Enzyme Diet™** later in this book, plus a variety of balanced simple meals to keep your taste buds tantalized and your palate titillated.

Reason #3.   Unrealistic Expectations

Dieters are among the most impatient people in the world. They want to lose some pounds and they want results now. That's why so many fad diets that promise inordinate guarantees become so notorious. *"Lose 30 pounds in 30 days." "Fit into the clothes you wore twenty years ago". "Get rid of those love handles fast." "Lose weight while you sleep."* You've seen the ads. You've heard the claims. You've watched the gimmicks. There are so many diet programs offering such dramatic results for so little effort and in so little time.

The gullible dieter who wants the easy way out and wants the 'quick fix' goes on some ridiculous diet, deceived into thinking that they'll be good for 'before and after pictures'. Every day, they're on the scales looking for change. They stand in front of the mirror, hoping to see a new body without the extra bulges. They'll do anything to realize their immediate goal, but their actions must produce immediate results. Soon their hopes are dashed. Even if they see some early weight loss due usually to loss of water, and maybe even loss of some lean mass as the body responds to the typical starvation diet, it never continues.   The weight reduction never lasts. Therefore, dieters with the most unreasonable expectations quit their program in disappointment. They give up either because they fail to see early results consistent with the exaggerated claims, or they get some early reduction that soon stops and even reverts. That's major anti-climax!

A great weight management program like **The Enzyme Diet™ Solution** will include a realistic strategy for weight loss. This will be appropriate for each individual and sustainable over the long haul.

Physiologically, a reduction of just a few pounds each week is near ideal, except perhaps for the more visible changes at the onset due more to water loss than actual fat. Those who are truly obese obviously have a lot more to lose and usually can do so more quickly.

Reason #4.   Poor Discipline

No matter how you look at it, anything in life that's worth having, being or doing, will demand a price. For the person who is overweight or even obese, it is certain that effective weight loss will require change: change of diet, change of self image, change of habits, change of lifestyle. Someone correctly observed that '*it is a form of insanity when one does the same old things, yet expects different results*'. Weight loss is no exception to the rule. To lose weight effectively and even moreso, to keep it off, you must exercise consistent discipline.

Many a dieter got started, but they had limited commitment to their goal. With loose attitudes, a tendency to laziness and poor self-control, they would not ... they could not ... follow through. They often cheated on their diet and they consistently excused their lethargy and inactivity as they warmed the sofa and took the path of least resistance. They even rationalized their situation. They blamed every causative factor they could imagine but themselves, and made themselves the mere victims who could do no better or be no thinner than their naturally fat bodies would allow. But even as they packed it in, they knew they were fooling nobody but themselves. You must remember that action produces results - only action, consistent action. Nothing less will do for the dieting routines and protocols that you need, to lead to effective weight loss.

The Enzyme Diet™ Solution is relatively simple and satisfying. It takes the hassle out of daily calorie-counting and the guess work out of balancing your daily menu for adequate nutrients. It becomes less of a burden and more of a delight as you see results.

Reason #5.   Self Image

Weight is really a personal thing. It is a characteristic that each person lives with - 24/7. Every waking moment you must contend with your body mass. There's no avoiding it. Even before you look into a mirror, you first look into your mind. You carry around a mental picture of yourself that supercedes every external presentation. You can see yourself even with your eyes closed. You intimately know that person projected onto your mental screen and you either like them or you don't. But there's no getting away from them. They even speak to you, in words of praise or condemnation. They affirm you or put you down. By the time you see reflections of your body mass in the bathroom mirror or on the weight scales, you only confirm what you already know deep inside.

To love yourself is of the highest priority. It gives inner peace and projects a confident gait and balance. Smiling comes easily. There is no need to be shy or to retreat.

To go on a diet or weight loss program does not require a hatred of self or even constant criticism of your present appearance. You can feel good, consider yourself to even look good, and yet see a need for improvement and change. Those who begin a diet with this affirmation of self, personal dignity and worth are likely to follow through. But if you really dislike yourself, or think of yourself as a failure, a slob or even a fat pig, it won't take long before you lose even the desire to change. Your inner self-image would then be constrained by your outward appearance, rather than vice versa.

You are only what you think you are. He or she who thinks they will fail, has already lost the battle with their weight. In fact, they often get bruised and battered in the process and their first failed attempt at weight loss can actually lead to weight gain because they simply fail to care anymore. They let themselves go and before they know it, matters can get out of hand. A cycle of failure and shame followed by careless-ness and indifference soon sets in. Too many dieters have slipped into this mental and emotional abyss that leads to increased obesity.

This can all be avoided. As part of **The Enzyme Diet™ Solution,** you will cultivate a healthy self image that accepts and affirms yourself for who you are. You will find reasons to take pride in where you are right now without denying your goal for effective change. You will appreciate the essential meaning and difference of 'being' and 'becoming'. You will even come to embrace the process of change. You'll find your mind taking essential control, even over your body. After all, real weight management is a mental process.

Reason #6.   Weight Plateau

I've worked with lots of people like the patient I'll call Cynara. She is an avid tennis player who breezed through menopause with very few symptoms that required any intervention. But in her early fifties, she noticed that she had gained an additional 25 pounds above the 130 pounds she had a decade earlier. It happened ever so slowly and she was able to maintain her game. She did not really care until one day she was at a ball game and met an old friend, Linda, whose kids grew up with hers. Linda was still the tall, slender person she remembered and without a word being said, Cynara felt suddenly obese. By the time she arrived home, she had resolved to go on a diet, which she did.

Cynara changed her entire household menu, stacked up with all the low calorie foods she could find and continued her tennis. She was delighted at first to see how easily she lost 11 pounds. It took only four weeks. But then for the next four months, nothing budged. She was 144, no more and no less. She hit a plateau and got stuck. She persisted a further two months, and no further change. When she came back to see me, I advised her that she may now be at her ideal weight and must stick to her maintenance program. But she was not satisfied. She wanted to go back to the 130 pounds, size eight that she vividly remembered. She intensified her tennis and even took up jogging but that still did not help. In time, she gave up her strict diet and slowly began to reintroduce her calorie-rich foods and to indulge her sweet tooth. She cared less now but she worried more. In time she began to skip her exercise routine and her lifestyle reverted to what she was like the year before. And so did her weight. By the time I saw her next, she was then weighing 156 pounds again. She had gone full circle.

You must know when your body is telling you something. If you do your best, your body will respond best. You would have done your best when you are able

> i.) to reduce your total body calories and still maintain your metabolism with adequate nutrients and supplementary enzymes, and
>
> ii.) to incorporate moderate exercise into your lifestyle.

All that and more is possible with **The Enzyme Diet™ Solution.** Having done that, you will do well as a dieter to remember the prayer of St. Francis:

> *Give me the courage to change the things that can be changed,*
> *Give me the patience to accept what cannot be changed,*
> *But most of all,*
> *Give me the wisdom to know the difference.*

Reason #7.   Side Effects

Weight loss is often a worthy goal. It is a healthy ideal in a culture where the tendency to obesity is so rampant. But like every other intervention you entertain, you must always do risk-benefit analysis. This will vary from one method to another. In the extreme, the guaranteed weight loss paradigm might be simply to seal the mouth with duct tape. You'll lose weight, no doubt about it. But you will lose much more than that. What that represents in the extreme is really similar to what many thousands of dieters do every day. They eliminate from their diet, essential nutrients, and then they add all types of unproven and unsafe ingredients and products. The net result is that they experience a number of undesirable symptoms that reflect nutritional inadequacy. This could be as mild as headaches, weakness, fatigue, irritability, nausea, gastric upset and the like. These are common effects with very low calorie diets where to reduce calories, one eliminates foods rich in essential nutrients.

But things could be much worse. Side effects from herbal products and diet pills like we have noted with Ma Huang and Fen-phen for example, can become more serious. So often the unsuspecting dieter who follows the latest diet craze, finds that they begin to experience the unexpected and unwanted consequences of their folly. Eventually, they smarten up and realize that it's not worth it.

Overweight and obesity are health challenges yes, but their management requires a method that is first **safe**, then effective and convenient. Nothing less will do and after reading about **The Enzyme Diet™ Solution**, certainly nothing else will do for you.

Reason #8.   Time Constraints

Speaking of diets being effective and convenient brings us to another important reason why diets usually fail. It's not so much the diet per se but the demands on the dieter in this fast and crazy culture. Life is hectic, too hectic. We rush from beating the rush hour traffic in the morning, to keeping up with information overload throughout the day, to responding to e-mails, voice mails and active family life in a day that has more labors than hours. Everybody is busy and nobody has time to eat, much less to cook, even less to shop. Dietary responsibility goes by the wayside.

It's hard to design a family menu, and even harder to stick to it.

So very often, eating out becomes the norm, if you can afford it. And you know that eating out is not a friend to effective dieting. Eating on the run becomes a way of life and there's enough fast food, convenience food and junk food to cut meal times to the nearest minute. The industry does everything conceivable to keep it so, leading to a dieter's nightmare. Diets usually call for lots of salads, fresh fruits and vegetables. But there's no time to choose and to chill, no time to chop or to chew. That's for the birds. Or is it?

Diets usually call for balanced meals but there's no time for planning and preparing. This is a convenient, calorie-rich culture even for conscious consumers. So dieters often give in and give up, and their diets sooner or later go the way of the dodo birds.

Does that sound something like you. If it does, you'll need **The Enzyme Diet™ Solution** for its convenience.

Reason #9.   Huge Expense

In a free-market economy where price is determined by laws of supply and demand, suppliers often extract what the market can bear. It's no surprise that with the extremely high demand for weight loss at almost any cost, those companies and individuals that deliver products and services in this industry, often capture more than a fair price for what they offer. Weight loss can be expensive. Professional weight loss centers and medical clinics can command hundreds of dollars per month for membership fees, counseling services, brand-name low-calorie foods, prepackaged meals, diet aids and supplements. Before you know it, you as a dieter can be out of pocket a few thousand dollars before you attain your elusive goal. Then if, as is often the case, you show rebound and fail on your maintenance program, you could be on the hook again for a few thousand more. Needless to say, that would make you think twice. That's the point at which many a dieter falls off the weight wagon and chooses to follow some cheap, quick-fix alternative.

But weight loss need not be that expensive a proposition. You will learn later that with **The Enzyme Diet™ Solution** there is a simple, relatively inexpensive and effective approach to weight loss that will in fact save you money, reduce your weight and improve your health, all at the same time. Keep reading.

Reason #10.   Vain Aesthetics

The last reason to be considered why dieters most often fail on their weight loss program is by no means the least. It goes back to the fundamental driving force behind their weight loss adventure in the first place. Obese individuals who have a lot to lose are most likely to see the biggest change in weight and appearance. That's great! Very encouraging. But on the other hand, the millions who are obsessed by the few extra pounds that threaten their bikini figure on the beach or embarrass them in the local gym or country club - they usually have a hard time getting to their 'ideal' weight and staying there. They want a diet to reduce and remodel their anatomy. But that's setting themselves up for disappointment. I beg your pardon, that's not the way to get a new figure or a new physique. Flat ab's, steel buns, firm biceps and quads, bulging chests and narrow waistlines come from genetic endowment, consistent physical work-outs and a lifetime of discipline. Who are you kidding if you expect a diet to create a new you, without the exercise, training, and let's face it, the fantastic gene pool? Nobody but yourself.

The Enzyme Diet™ Solution   program will allow you to become physically the best that you can be. You are your greatest asset but you must become your own greatest fan.

So give yourself a shake and let's get down to business. Let's explore the real root of your weight problem. What makes you overweight? What can you change and how can you go about doing that? Then, what can't you change and how do you go about accepting, then affirming, and finally applauding that?

We begin at the fundamental weight paradigm - the calorie (energy) balance equation.

You Can't Avoid
THE CALORIE EQUATION

There is a fundamental law of science that appears incontrovertible in a closed system. It is called the First Law of Thermodynamics which could be simply stated as *Energy is neither created nor destroyed.* Most children in school will learn that Einstein discovered - a long time ago, it seems now - that energy and matter are interconvertible. So food is chemical energy locked up, waiting to be released.

What this means when applied to weight and dietary intake is that the human body shifts from its normal state of equilibrium (called homeostasis) when energy in the form of food is consumed. Approximately 10% of this energy is used in the process of digestion, transport and deposition of nutrients at their destination inside the cells of the body. The remaining bulk of this energy is either utilized or stored. This can be expressed in a single calorie (energy) balance equation:

$$\begin{array}{cccc} \text{Calories} & & \text{Calories for} & = & \text{Calories} & + & \text{Calories} \\ \text{In Food} & - & \text{Food Processing} & & \text{Utilized} & & \text{Stored} \end{array}$$

The fraction that is utilized, is actually converted (burned up) as the energy that fuels all the processes taking place inside the body: some to produce heat (thermogenesis); some to affect chemical changes like protein synthesis and thousands of other complex reactions (metabolism); and some to permit all forms of physical activity (exercise). This too can be expressed as a simple equation:

$$\begin{array}{cccc} \text{Calories} & = & \text{Calories for} & + & \text{Calories for} & + & \text{Calories for} \\ \text{Utilized} & & \text{Adaptation} & & \text{Metabolism} & & \text{Exercise} \end{array}$$

Normal thermogenesis allows the body to adapt (hence, calories for adaptation) and maintain a fairly stable temperature of 37 degrees Celsius or 98.4 degrees Fahrenheit, even though the ambient temperature of the external environment is usually much lower. The energy utilized when the body is at rest (just as you are now, resting perhaps and reading this book), refers to the Resting Metabolic Rate. When exercise is included, the total energy utilized refers to the overall metabolic rate. The resting metabolic rate is normally about 60-75% of the total energy you would utilize (burn) each day. Exercise represents the minor (about 20-30%) component but as we shall see, its value lies in the fact that it is a variable component (remember the prayer of St. Francis).

You can actually have your metabolic rate measured by a sophisticated apparatus called a *Metabolic Cart*. It actually measures the amount of oxygen you consume at rest, but this is not commonly available. A good approximation comes from determining your lean muscle mass. Actually, the way this is done is to measure your body fat level by a *Bioelectric Impedance Meter*. These are available in some doctors' clinics or health clubs and you might even find one to purchase at your local department store, if you were so inclined. To measure fat, the impedance meter sends a very small electric current through your body and the resistance is determined. Since muscle conducts electricity while fat does not, you can derive the amount of your lean muscle mass. From this you simply calculate your metabolic rate as follows: Each pound of lean muscle mass burns typically 14 calories per day. If you are a woman with say 100 pounds of lean muscle mass, your basic metabolic rate is therefore about 1400 calories per day. If you are male with say 150 pounds of lean muscle mass, you will likewise burn about 2100 calories per day. You should appreciate this concept of lean muscle mass because as you lose weight, you want always to be aware of what changes are really taking place. In other words, aim to lose fat and preserve your lean mass.

Now, let's briefly consider the important role of exercise. Is it really important for dieters? The answer is unequivocally, yes! Exercise has both short term and long term consequences. In the short term, it increases the amount of energy utilized significantly, so that for the same energy intake as food, there is less residual to be stored. That follows directly from the calorie (energy) balance equation we just described above.

In the short term, low end aerobic exercise is best as you start out. Especially so, if you have had a sedentary lifestyle of late. More particularly, walking slowly and comfortably or recreational swimming are perhaps the best and most efficient ways to get moving. Why? Because when you walk or swim like this, about 60% of the total energy that you burn comes directly from fat storage. In addition, you can do this for extended periods. On the contrary, fast (demanding), exhaustive exercise will utilize energy stored as muscle glycogen first. Nature tends to reserve and preserve fat as long term storage for a rainy day.

This may be the best way to start out, but it is obviously not the ultimate in exercise. After you become physically active again, you will need to increase your intensity, and interval training will be most important. Both low-intensity for fat-burning and high intensity for calorie burning are needed. In reality, although a greater percentage of calories used during exercise at low intensity is from fat, the actual amount of fat burned is about the same as that burned during a high intensity workout.

In the long term, anaerobic exercise (i.e. high intensity, for short periods of time), such as body building or weight (resistance) training - as well as more active sports like cycling and hiking - will all build muscle which increases lean body mass. This in turn will increase the resting metabolic rate and increase energy utilization. There'll be much more on that later.

Dieters are quick to focus on the other big parameter in the calorie balance equation: the amount of calories consumed as food. Almost all diets target low-calories as the bottom line. The fewer calories you take in, the less you will have to store. Therefore, obesity is explained often by calorie accounting. For example, if you eat a typical 2500 calorie diet and only burn 2000 calories per day, you will store an excess of 500 calories per day or 3500 calories each week. That is the equivalent amount of energy for one pound of fat, so you should gain about one pound per week. That could be 50 pounds in one year, all other things being equal! On the other hand, if you consume only 1500 calories per day on some diets and still burn 2000 calories, you will have a net deficit of 500 calories per day or 3500 calories per week. You should then expect to lose one pound per week or four pounds per month, on average. No wonder, the calorie counters have a field day. It's no wonder so many dieters are going crazy with arithmetic.

But whoever said that life was simple and straightforward like that. The truth is, it's not. There are variations between individuals because of our genetic makeup for one thing and besides that, all calories are not equal. Inside the body, with all its regulatory control mechanisms, some calories are more 'equal' than others.

Addressing the **hereditary** issue, we know that identical twins raised apart from each other, tend to have very similar weights. In other words, their common genes seem to have a dominant role. But on the contrary, fraternal twins do not have exactly the same genetic make up. In this case, they can show very different responses when fed the same large amounts of food over say three months. Some might gain a mere ten pounds, while their corresponding twins might gain twenty pounds or more. This is a clear reflection of the importance of genes influencing obesity. It is also clear that obese children, even if removed from their childhood environment, tend to become obese adults. That is not an unequivocal genetic consequence in this case, but it is at least consistent.

This genetic component and the fact that calories are not created equal, brings us to examine next the concept of metabolic rate more closely and then the issue of internal regulatory hormones. So we first come to what is known as set point theory.

~

Set Points are NOT Set In Stone

Most weight control experts and other professionals have concluded that the overall level of body weight and the relative amount of body fat that each individual displays is affected by a number of different factors or conditions. It is not as simple as the calorie (energy) balance equation above would imply. That would make weight loss a simple product of applied arithmetic. But we know that is not the case, especially when we observe the almost ubiquitous tendency to yo-yo dieting. No sooner do you lose some weight, then something seems to happen to work against your best efforts and back it comes. How many times have you heard that lament? You've probably experienced the same thing.

Medical researchers at the Laboratory of Human Behavior and Metabolism at Rockefeller University in New York have advanced a theory which has gained support and with some good evidence, to provide a new understanding if not first an explanation, of this yo-yo dieting phenomenon. Dr. Rudolph Leibel, one of the lead scientists, posed the question in the title of a paper in 1990: "Is obesity due to a heritable difference in 'set point' for adiposity?" [1] What he was implying was that each individual might be biologically and genetically determined to weigh within a certain weight range. In other words, people tend to end up at a weight that is specific for them. You have a weight range, within a few pounds, which is healthy and normal for you. **This range is called your 'set point'.**

If you just ate normally when you were hungry, stopped when

you were full and exercised in moderation, you would arrive at a weight inside a small range that would be just healthy and normal for you. Whenever you attempt to step outside that range, your body would react. A defensive mechanism would set in. If for example, you try to lose weight and you begin to succeed so that you fall below your 'normal and healthy' range (your set-point), your body would react by decreasing your metabolism and increasing your hunger. That's how the theory goes. By slowing the metabolic rate, you would burn fewer calories to avoid the apparent 'starvation' that your body thinks is imminent. Your metabolism could actually decrease by as much as 40%. You would develop obsessional thinking about food, weight and hunger. Your hunger itself would become more intense and last longer as the body resists any significant deviation from your 'set point'. This can account for the bingeing habits that dieters fall into for sure. In addition, you may start to sleep more and your body temperature could fall slightly. Some women can lose enough weight to cause their menstrual cycle to be interrupted as their reproductive system shuts down. In a way, that's all unnatural. It is life in reverse.

What is more, your body thinks that it really is going to starve. So, guess what? It does the unthinkable. It tries to preserve its valuable energy stores without which it cannot survive. It preserves …fat! After all, fat is its most energy-dense reserve, so it becomes most valuable. We'll come back to this, but suffice it to note here that **the body preserves fat by increasing the activity of the enzymes that synthesize fat for storage and decreasing the activity of fat digestive enzymes.** Just note this crucial role of enzymes.

I am sure that you are beginning to suspect a major role for **The Enzyme Diet™** already. But let's not get ahead of ourselves.

Dr. Leibel and his colleagues at Rochester have published papers to demonstrate clinically what we just described as 'changes in energy expenditure resulting from altered body weight.' [2] They examined the effects of experimentally altering the weights of otherwise healthy, volunteer subjects under controlled conditions. They showed that any attempt to maintain a reduced or elevated body weight was generally associated with compensatory changes in each subject's energy utilization. This in turn opposed the effort to achieve prolonged weight loss or weight gain. The tendency was always to return the subject to his or her initial stable weight.

Set points vary for each individual. Therefore, it would be unwise for you to simply go by the average weight charts commonly found in popular magazines, diet books or doctors' offices. Your body will be most healthy and truly normal when your weight is in the set point range determined by your own genetic makeup. Somewhere in your brain, it is believed - probably in the region of the hypothalamus which acts like a high level, central-control for your hormone regulation - is *a fat control center* that literally sets your ideal weight at any given age and stage of your life. This unconscious and automatic device continually assesses your body's inventory of stored fat and takes steps to adjust it like any good manager does.

This is all good news and bad news at the same time. The good news for the person who is overweight or even obese is naturally, that you cannot just be blamed for being some kind of gluttonous couch-potato - like it's all your fault. That's clearly not so. The bad news is a bit worse. You may actually be programmed to be something other than the lean sterotypic model that you or somebody you know wishes you were.

You've heard a bit of good news and some bad news. Now let me share with you as Paul Harvey would say, *'the rest of the story'*. It's better news:

Your set-point can be changed!

Let's consider, for example, the work of Dr. Roland Weinsier, Director of the Clinical Nutrition Research Center at the University of Alabama, Birmingham, Alabama. He reported that in his research, he found that formerly overweight people have metabolisms similar to those who have never been overweight. In a study published in the *American Journal of Clinical Nutrition* in November, 2000, he reported that over a four year period, he followed 24 overweight women who dieted, and compared them with another 24 never obese, control subjects (3). The study found that although resting metabolic rate fell while the women were on a diet, it returned to normal when their food intake also returned to normal. In the dieting group, 85% of the women regained much of the weight lost. They lost an average of 30 pounds on their low calorie diets. However, variations in their resting metabolic rate did not predict the amount of weight they regained. That was a function more of their individual dietary and exercise habits in their normal environments. Factors other than an abnormal metabolic rate must be responsible for the tendency to regain weight. Failure to lose weight permanently is not just due to a shift in metabolism per se, but an inability to continue on a well designed weight loss program.

The American environment is the direct opposite. That's why we find it so hard to maintain weight loss. There's just too much external attraction (calorie-rich food) and distraction (passive entertainment). We therefore put in too much energy as food calories and tend to work off not quite enough. The set point is therefore only a part of the whole story.

There is in fact, a new variation of this control theory, now called the "*Settling Point Theory*". It forces us to take the external environment and lifestyle into account. It upstages the Set Point Theory by pointing to the recent epidemic of overweight and obesity that is clearly documented right across the American population. Surely, there must be something in the area of dieting that is at fault. They point a straight finger at the suspect and they even rush to judgement. Fat is the culprit!

Some people have fat cells that produce more *enzymes to digest fat* than others. Those that produce less of these enzymes, store more fat. But that extra fat subsequently influces the production of more enzymes, to digest more fat and therefore store less. This type of feedback leads to a settling point or equilibrium, influenced by the fat intake but limited by the genetic expression of **fat enzymes**.

The bottom line here must be that you cannot throw up your hands or become resigned to some kind of genetic determinism or fate in the face of the silent epidemic of overweight and obesity. You must take responsibility. All the factor interests like industry, government, media, educators, etc. that create the environment to make weight management such a huge challenge, must also take responsibility. But, in the end, it is still bad diets, poor choices, sedentary lifestyles and lack of discipline that ultimately cause healthful dieting to fail.

You will learn in this book that **The Enzyme Diet™ Solution** is a new paradigm for treating obesity effectively. Perhaps the Set Point Theory gave rise to the Settling Point Theory only to give rise now to the **Enzyme Theory**, or the **Enzyme Index**, or the **Enzyme Quotient**, whatever you prefer.

Any sensible weight loss program must take this set point hypothesis seriously. The body will react to change. If you cut back, it will slow down. But the cause is not lost. Both diet and exercise can directly influence your set point or your body's acceptable level of fat storage. On the downside, if you continue to eat lots of fat and sweets, your set point will rise, your appetite will increase and you'll gain more weight. You'll then perhaps try yet another low calorie diet and your body will over-react by slowing your metabolism and giving you hunger pangs. That will constrain you to resume binge eating of more fats and sugars - and you'll be back where you started. It becomes a vicious cycle! This is the common pattern for millions who go on a diet each year.

A more rational approach will aim to maintain adequate cellular nutrition and active metabolism so the cycle is broken and you could be free to lose weight and still be satisfied and healthy. That's exactly the experience with **The Enzyme Diet™ Solution**.

In addition, there is no getting away from exercise, no matter what diet you choose. Physical activity is the prime natural influence that seems capable of resetting the set point. How or why this is so, is not entirely clear. But exercise does appear to help keep whatever the set point system is, functioning properly. You take the first step by getting up and getting out, and getting on the walking trails or the treadmill, and getting into the swimming pool, and your body will reward your natural efforts by improving efficiency, turning on your 'after burners' and dropping your set point. You meet your end of the bargain, and your body will not disappoint you as long as you persist and maintain the discipline of healthy dieting and moderate exercise. Therefore, put your set point to work for you.

It is still true that your set point is primarily determined by your genes. However, that set point is not set in stone. Your genes represent only one factor among others. In fact, too many people confuse their genes with their hormones. But you cannot blame your hormones either.

Don't Blame Your Hormones

At a physiological level, the body utilizes very small amounts of circulating molecules that are empowered to control most biological functions. These hormones operate in a hierarchy of responsibility and authority, with some central control by the hypothalamic area of the brain. They turn-on and turn-off systems. They speed up and slow down others. They trigger build up and initiate breakdown. They regulate cycles, from daily sleeping and waking, to monthly reproductive preparation, to the entire lifespan itself. They prepare the body for fight or flight and yes, they dictate how, when, where, why and what we do with the food we eat. Specifically, they impact when we consume food, what we digest, how much we absorb, what we utilize and how much we store. Therefore, the weight we have is clearly affected by our hormones. Of special importance to us, in terms of weight management, are the following four hormones: *insulin, thyroxine, estrogen* and a newcomer to this area called *leptin*.

Insulin

Insulin is clearly one of the most powerful and efficient substances that the body uses to control the use, distribution and storage of energy in the form of the simple sugar, glucose. Glucose is the basic unit of currency in the body's energy economy. It fuels all the operating systems, including the highest control centers of the brain. In fact, a supply of glucose to the brain is perhaps rivaled only by oxygen in importance. The body therefore does everything to preserve an adequate supply of glucose to fuel its entire operation and it does so in desperation under all conditions.

The principle source of glucose is derived from the daily diets. All the major classes of foods become sources of glucose after digestion and assimilation. Simple sugars are absorbed from the gut quickly and easily. More complex *carbohydrates* are broken down to form simple sugars and are then absorbed. *Fats* are digested into free-fatty-acids and glycerol for absorption. The free fatty acids are a source of energy and in starvation, glycerol is converted to glucose. The third major component of food is *protein* and that too is digested into its constituent amino acids for absorption and they can be converted in a complex sequence of reactions to form glucose. Glucose then is the common energy currency.

If glucose is the common energy currency of the body, then insulin acts like the central banker overseeing the money supply and approving, or even facilitating, every transaction. In fact, there are two critical functions it performs exceptionally well.

First, insulin reduces the level of glucose in your bloodstream by channeling it into the various body tissues on demand for short term use, or by storing it as fat. Secondly, it inhibits the conversion of body fat back into glucose, thereby protecting its inventory or reserve for less prosperous times. Fat is like the treasury, the storage vault or central bank and insulin is very protective. It is kept in check and on its toes as it were, by opposing counter-regulatory hormones - especially glucagon, adrenocorticoids and adrenalin. But insulin still dominates.

So far, so good.

Insulin however, has been implicated by some as the major culprit in promoting obesity. You will recognize these advocates from Chapter 2 as promoters of some popular diets like *The Atkins Diet, The Carbohydrate Addict Diet, Sugar Busters* and *The Zone Diet.* These prominent diet gurus make a case that does not really stand up to serious scrutiny. They associate overweight and obesity with high insulin levels caused by high levels of carbohydrate, including all kinds of sugar, in the diet. Their argument has not found scientific acceptance because the evidence is to the contrary. But let's see the argument they use.

The insulin hypothesis goes something like this. When you eat carbohydrate (especially sugar in all its forms), the rapid rise of glucose in your blood causes the pancreas to secrete more insulin. This rush of insulin causes the glucose to be converted into glycogen first and when these storage sites are full, the remaining glucose is stored as triglyceride or plain fat. Simply put, insulin produces fat. This all arises from the sugar boom or carbohydrate addiction. Proteins and fats in the diet do not cause any similar insulin surge.

Even worse than that, the theory goes, as fat increases, the action of insulin becomes less effective and so to get the job done, more insulin is produced. They argue that the receptors for insulin on the surface of cells become blocked, hence those cells do not function properly either. The term '*insulin resistance*' is then used to account for the over production of insulin. As more and more insulin is produced, the pancreas assumes more and more of a burden until it begins to feel the strain and Type 2 (non-insulin dependent) diabetes is observed. If the pancreas deteriorates further until it is exhausted and can no longer produce enough insulin, insulin injections would then be required for survival.

Back to the question of obesity itself. This theory of hyperinsulinism as a major cause of obesity even accounts for some obese behavior patterns. When lots of insulin is produced in response to a fast rise in blood glucose, the quick response in susceptible individuals causes the glucose to be utilized or stored quickly and the blood sugar levels fall and become abnormally low. This leads to symptoms of tiredness, weakness, irritability and hunger! The tendency is to eat more - usually more of the same, to produce more symptoms - and the pattern becomes addictive behavior which accentuates the weight problem!

The above hypothesis might sound good on the surface but it does not concur with the facts. It's a case of the proverbial chicken-and-egg. Many independent studies have shown that high insulin levels do not cause weight gain. In fact, they get the whole issue of diabetes, insulin-resistance and obesity, the wrong way round. As we pointed out in the last chapter, insulin resistance does not lead to obesity. Rather, it is the *obesity that leads to insulin resistance* that favors diabetes. Just think! In clinical practice, the doctor advises the diabetic patient to lose weight. If they do, they can often reduce their insulin or cut back on their diabetic pills. Notice the intervention. You do not target the diabetes to influence the obesity. You *address the obesity as the primary associated cause*, in order to target the secondary insulin dependence or the need for hypoglemics by the diabetic patient. All the evidence shows that effective weight reduction in obese diabetics tends to reduce the requirements for insulin or diabetic pills. That's the real situation.

Yet there is a redeeming feature in all this. The emphasis on avoiding simple sugars is good, for more reasons than one. The shift to more complex carbohydrates with their lower glycemic index is very wise, healthy and less fattening. However, the caution to achieve a balance that includes adequate proteins and fat as well as carbohydrates, in the overall diet, is certainly consistent with the best of nutritional knowledge. '*Man shall not live by bread* (carbs) *alone*' is both a spiritual and practical truism.

So let's choose to eat right and leave the insulin alone. That is not the culprit per se. Insulin is an intrinsic regulatory hormone, essential to life, and responsive to your nutritional and other lifestyle patterns. A balanced dietary approach will negate whatever residual insulin anxiety you may have.

The Enzyme Diet™ Solution will help you to achieve that balance.

Thyroxine

Let me tell you about another patient of mine. We'll call her Sabrina. I first met her when she was in her early twenties. At that time she was a happy mother of two small children and worked as an airline attendant, flying all over the world for a major airline. She was of average build and about 5'5" tall. She was an avid pianist and loved to dance. By all reports from her husband, she was often the life of the party whenever she was out socially.

By her late twenties, I noticed on routine examination that her weight began to creep upward. Over the period of one year, she added some six to ten pounds to her earlier stable weight of 123 pounds. During that time, she began to complain of fatigue and dry skin but no immediate action was indicated. By the following year, those symptoms had worsened and what triggered my attention and follow up was when she complained of being bothered by the cold, while others about her seemed quite comfortable. Her menstrual flow increased. Her weight continued to creep upward past 135 pounds, her hair became slightly coarse and her voice tended to be often a bit hoarse. She was not feeling her normal energetic self. In fact, she was entering a borderline depression. She wanted some time off which I approved and focused more definitively on possible physiological causes for her complaints.

To jump to my later diagnostic conclusion, Sabrina was found to have low levels of the hormone thyroxine in her blood. Her thyroid gland was underactive, even though it was not palpable. She had no family history of goitre but I was able to do further thyroid function tests on her, including measuring her thyroid stimulating hormones. I found that she had a primary disease of the thyroid gland called Hashimoto's Thyroiditis, a benign auto-immune condition. I was able to treat her with small doses of levothyroxine replacement. She is still on that drug today and her thyroxine levels are continually monitored every few months. The good news is that all her symptoms were reversed, including a restoration of her agile 125 pound frame with the help of **The Enzyme Diet™**. She is still the life of her party now, at least when she is not flying the skies somewhere or other.

Sabrina's case illustrates so well a fairly common condition in the general population. Thyroxine replacement is a very common prescription drug in many doctors' offices. However, underactive thyroid is not a common cause of obesity - far from it. It accounts for less than 1%

of overweight conditions and makes at most a mild contribution to obesity.

How does thyroxine affect a person's weight? The thyroxine circulates in the blood and becomes attached to the special thyroid hormone receptors in the nuclei of cells. This ultimately effects the synthesis of proteins inside those cells. As such then, thyroxine becomes a trigger or boost to cellular metabolism. When the level of this hormone becomes relatively low, the body's metabolic rate slows down. If we go back to the *calorie balance equation* discussed earlier, this has the effect of burning less calories and therefore storing more. However, it is not uncommon to find overweight and obese patients who have underactive thyroid but whose weight reflects other concommitant factors. You can't just blame a sluggish thyroid for a bulging body, a depressed personality and an inactive lifestyle. If you ever put thyroxine in the trial box and give it its day in obesity court, the judge and jury would most likely use the evidence to give a unanimous verdict: *Not Guilty*!

The Enzyme Diet™ Solution will still make sense, even for those dieters who have to supplement with levothyroxine for whatever reason.

Estrogen

So if it's not insulin per se, and if it's not the thyroid, what else can you find to blame? Many women conclude that it's all because of their estrogen. **It's a woman thing**, they say. Just consider the facts.

At puberty, when estrogen levels begin to increase, even the skinny adolescent girl starts to put on weight as she develops her feminine characteristics - curves and all. If she goes on oral contraceptives - which are a form of estrogen - she will often observe that weight increase tends to be a side effect of the pill. Then with marriage may come pregnancy and later breast feeding. As the hormones surge, the fetus grows and her weight is monitored at every prenatal visit. She watches the scales. After delivery, it is not uncommon for her to struggle to regain her original size and shape. That often turns out to be a losing battle. Those child-bearing hips tend to hang around and after the healthy experience of breastfeeding, there is often a visible price. When the children are grown, then comes menopause. No surprise there. The hormones are all over the map and the general tendency is for estrogen levels to fall off as the ovaries begin to fail. But fat (adipose tissue) is a source of estrogen synthesis and storage, so it is not surprising that her body partly compensates for the ovaries by increasing fat. That's her late middle age spread. Later with decreased estrogen, muscle atrophy sets in, the skin loses its elasticity and loose fat becomes more prominent. No wonder many a woman retorts, *'It's my hormones, stupid.* Blame those ovaries. Blame the children. Blame the drug companies. Blame my doctor. Blame anyone but me.'

Nobody can deny the important role of sex hormones in women (and men too!) throughout the life cycle. But we can deny that overweight and obesity in women can be accounted for or excused just by hormones, as if those endogenous hormones are rate-limiting in terms of any weight changes. If you are a woman, it is still very much your personal responsibility to look after yourself. You can control your diet, engage in moderate physical activity, cultivate a healthy lifestyle and enjoy only modest weight gain as you grow to full maturity and enjoy the best that life has to offer. **The Enzyme Diet™ Solution** can work for you too.

Leptin and More

Insulin, thyroxine, estrogen - these were quick and easy suspects to bear the blame for this seemingly natural tendency, at least in some significant segments of the population, to put on weight: more weight than the rest of us. But then, such well known hormones have been tried and found not guilty as charged. They may be accomplices to the genetic conspiracy but they could not be held primarily responsible.

So the search continues.

A major break in the case was suspected a few years ago with the discovery of a brand new hormone. Another group of researchers at Rockefeller University in New York, led by a molecular geneticist, Dr. Jeffrey Friedman, found that fat cells in mice produce a hormone which actually causes fat to melt away (4). It was labeled leptin, a name derived from the Greek word *leptos*, which translates *thin*.

These researchers used genetic engineering to develop mice that did not have the known gene for making this hormone. These mice turned out to have huge appetites. They could hardly stop eating and they put on weight like crazy. They were then injected with the missing hormone and by this single intervention, they were made to lose one third of the weight they had gained.

Mice tend to behave usually like 'little people,' so this created a lot of excitement among other researchers in the field. Unfortunately though, tests on humans found that almost all obese subjects actually had normal levels of this newly discovered leptin hormone.

Nevertheless, leptin must somehow be a key player in the delicate balance of energy utilization and storage in the body. It influences the amount of food we have the urge to eat and the amount of energy we choose to burn as heat. It would appear that as fat storage increases, more leptin is produced to reverse the trend. The mode of action is probably at the control center in the hypothalamus. However, those people who are predisposed to gain weight develop a form of leptin resistance. As they gain weight, their fat cells produce more leptin, but the hypothalamus becomes more insensitive. Eventually, their control center misreads the drop in leptin that accompanies weight loss as a signal for semi-starvation and slows the metabolism. Hence, the tendency to rebound weight gain and the persistence of that yo-yo cycle that every dieter loves to hate.

But with this announcement, the pace of the investigation quickened and there was a rush of new reports of hormone regulation of appetite (to control caloric intake) and hormone effects in thermogenesis (to control caloric expenditure).

The bottom line is that there must be a number of interconnected hormonal and even neural pathways to-and-from the hypothtalamus that provide delicate regulation and feedback inhibition to maintain stable body weight even when the typical person can consume and expend about one million calories per year. We are just beginning to understand this very complex system.

No matter what turn this hormone pursuit takes in the next few years, we can be sure that genetic determination is not the ultimate reason for obesity. Some people are clearly more predisposed and susceptible, yes. There is a tendency for weight problems to run in families. But how can one account for the rising incidence across the board? Even in the same individual, there are patterns of weight gain and loss that clearly reflect the impact of lifestyle and environment. Diet is central and dieting makes consummate sense, if the right type of diet could be followed, and in the context of a balanced and comprehensive program. **The Enzyme Diet™ Solution** makes a prime candidate.

As a summary to this problem of overweight and obesity in general, let us now look at what constitutes the essential characteristics of what conceivably could be an ideal weight loss diet.

The Ideal Weigh Loss Diet

Characteristic #1.   **Controlled Calories**

No matter how you come at it, every weight loss diet must obey the *Law of Conservation of Energy*. The *calorie balance equation* is explicit that your body will store the energy it does not use, as fat. Normal fat metabolism will only lead to a reduction if there is a higher demand for energy as calories than the amount being consumed. Therefore, diets designed for weight loss must limit caloric intake.

The question then arises: How many calories should you have on a daily basis?

The average adult in America typically consumes about 2000-3000 calories each day when weight considerations are not in the picture. Obviously, athletes and body builders for example, usually consume more, whereas seniors and sick patients tend to eat less. But, by and large, anything around 2500 calories a day is certainly in the healthy range for most people without a weight challenge.

It is generally agreed that the normal person could *get by* on a total daily diet of about 1100-1200 calories, if they made very careful food choices. They could do this by design, probably for a limited time, without complication and without any form of medical supervision. This is the reasonable lower limit to avoid any major changes in physiology. Such minimum caloric intake just affords the essential amounts of energy for normal activity. Less than this would cause your body to switch over to a 'starvation' mode and the side effects and potential complications could then set in. That's when you could begin to suffer from fatigue, weakness, headaches, stomach cramps, and the like. You then lose weight and possibly much more too. You want to avoid that for sure.

Under medical supervision, the experts go down as low as 500-600 calories per day for more rapid weight loss in their more obese patients. These very low calorie diets (VLCDs) could lead to clinical changes that need professional management and are not designed for the general unsupervised public. In any case, such patients are monitored. Their diets tend to be short term (weeks to months), with responsive intervention to be taken whenever clinically indicated.

Characteristic #2.   Adequate Nutrients

Food supplies energy to the body but it must also supply much more. Food proteins contain *essential* amino acids that are used to synthesize thousands of different proteins in your body with a vast array of different specialized functions. The term 'essential' implies that of the 22 known amino acid building blocks that constitute all human proteins, some 13 or 14 of them cannot be made or converted by your body. They must be supplied in your diet or your body would not be able to make most of the proteins that it depends on for survival and health. Imagine an automobile assembly line with some of the car parts missing in inventory. That shuts the entire plant down. Similarly, any and every diet, designed for weight loss or not, must have adequate supplies of essential amino acids in food proteins for cellular protein synthesis.

For your general information, you can estimate your own intrinsic need for proteins by simple arithmetic. Most normal adults require an amount of daily protein in grams equal to their weight in kilograms multiplied by 0.8. So if you are now 80kg (176lbs), you typically need 80 x 0.8 = 64 grams (2 oz.) of protein daily. However, when following a calorie restricted diet, the need for protein intake is increased, since some amino acids are used for energy.

Just as for amino acids, there are also *essential* vitamins, *essential* minerals and essential fatty acids and fiber. These are nutrients that must also be obtained from your diet as regular foods or supplements. In general, fruits and vegetables are rich in vitamins and minerals; dairy products are a good source of calcium; lean meats provide iron as well as protein; whole grains and cereals are full of complex carbohydrate and essential fiber.

Table 3 lists some selected food sources and daily recommendations for essential vitamins and minerals. Essential fatty acids and fiber will be covered later in Chapter 6.

Table 3.   Essential Vitamins and Minerals

Vitamins	RDA/AI mg/d	Some Selected Food Sources
Biotin	0.03	Liver, smaller amounts in fruits and meat
Choline	425-550	Milk, liver, eggs, peanuts
Folate	0.4-0.6	Enriched cereal grains, dark leafy vegs, some breads
Niacin	14-16	Meat, fish, poultry, enriched breads
Pantothenic acid	5	Chicken, beef, potatoes, oats, tomato, liver
Riboflavin (B2)	1.1-1.3	Organ meats, milk, breads, fortified cereals
Thiamin (B1)	1.1-1.2	Whole grain products, breads, cereals
Vitamin A	0.7-0.9	Liver, dairy products, fish
Vitamin B6	1.3-1.7	Fortified cereals, organ meats, soya meat substitutes
Vitamin B12	0.0024	Fortified cereals, meat, fish, poultry
Vitamin C	75-90	Citrus, tomatoes, potatoes, sprouts, cauliflower
Vitamin D	0.005-0.010	Fish liver oils
Vitamin E	15	Vegetable oils, grains, nuts, fruits, veg., meats
Vitamin K	0.090-0.120	Green vegetables, brussel sprouts, cabbage

Minerals

Minerals	RDA/AI mg/d	Some Selected Food Sources
Calcium	1200	Dairy, corn, tofu, kale, broccoli
Iron	8-18	Meats, fruits, vegetables, fortified breads and grains
Chromium	0.020-0.035	Some cereals, meats, poultry, fish
Copper	0.9	Organ meats, seafoods, nuts, seeds
Fluoride	3-4	Fluoridated water, teas, marine fish
Iodine	0.015	Marine origin, iodized salt
Magnesium	300-420	Green leafy vegetables, nuts, meat
Manganese	1.8-2.3	Nuts, legumes, tea, whole grains
Molybdenum	0.045	Legumes, grain products, nuts
Phosphorus	700-1250	Dairy, peas, meat, eggs
Selenium	0.055	Organ meats, seafood, some plants
Nickel, Boron	N/A	Various
Silicon, Vanadium	N/A	Various

An unbalanced or inadequate diet will starve your cells of their essential input. This would derail their metabolism, limit growth and repair, and reduce their capacity for efficient immune response. Sick cells make up sick organs that cause bodies to get sick and eventually die. Therefore cellular nutrition is the fundamental basis of all health. Any responsible weight loss diet must promote your cellular health and must deliver to you an adequate smorgasbord of all the essential nutrients.

That's what **The Enzyme Diet**™ does.

Characteristic #3.   Metabolic Boost

We have already noted that the normal response to weight loss is for the body to slow down its metabolism to reduce energy expenditure. This alters the body's physiology to the extent that dieting can become counter productive. In some cases, not only does the dieter regain the weight lost when any kind of normal diet is restored (by design or even by default), but over time, additional weight may be gained and lean muscle mass can be replaced by storage fat.

The ideal weight loss diet must address this issue. Somehow the body must be encouraged or stimulated to maintain near normal metabolic rates. As we will see in the next major section (Part II) when we present **The Enzyme Diet**™ as the best solution for effective and sustainable weight loss, there are some innovative approaches to doing just that. We will learn that the forgotten key to metabolism is the ubiquitous action of metabolic enzymes. They are the indispensable workforce for everything that the cell does. Nutrients are derived from food by the effective action of digestive enzymes that break down complex macromolecules into simple constituents for absorption and assimilation. Further, by original formulation it is possible to guarantee more efficient delivery of those very nutrients to the cells where they are destined to prime the unceasing intracellular biological activity. All these considerations are exploited in practical ways in the original formulation of **The Enzyme Diet**™.

But we are again getting ahead of ourselves. That's the subject of Part II where we will actually present the *solution* to this nagging weight loss challenge.

Characteristic #4.   Enough Variety

Food is pleasure. It appeals to your senses and surrounded as you are by such an abundance of enticing delights, to attempt any dietary program that is too restrictive and even downright boring to any normal healthy person, is to set yourself up for regression and disappointment.

The ideal weight loss diet must provide for you a variety of meals on the total menu. It must give you a variety of choices that caters to your peculiar tastes and preferences. With constant appeal from advertising, shopping displays, the aromas of fine cuisine and sumptuous desserts everywhere, how can anyone survive on a monotonous repetition of the same limited fare that some diets promote? Variety implies variety of taste and color, variety of food presentation and flavor, plus a variety of snacks and treats for your own personal impulsive satisfaction - all that and more.

As you will see later, **The Enzyme Diet™ Solution** again does exactly that. Each day the diet can be varied to satisfy your taste and desire for indulgence. Variety is more than the spice of life, it is the hook of the ideal weight loss diet to keep you interested enough to follow the plan, and committed enough to follow through to lasting results.

Characteristic #5.   Convenient Satisfaction

In the hectic pace of today's lifestyle and culture, you probably demand so much more of yourself and others around you. You want to be productive, efficient and reliable. You have no time to waste on non-essentials and trivia. Work is demanding, family is consuming and even when you find personal time in your guarded private space, chores become burdensome. There is no room for a diet that requires you to make major shopping expeditions to find exotic ingredients. Meals should be relatively quick and easy to prepare - not necessarily delicate and fancy. There's nothing like finding what you need immediately at hand, putting ingredients together simply but tastefully, and then quickly and quietly enjoying a smooth, delightful drink, or the healthy low calorie snack, or one balanced and attractive rainbow meal. This is 21st century living. This sounds just like **The Enzyme Diet™ Solution**.

At the end of the day, the ideal weight loss diet should deliver to you enough nutrition and bulk to create a feeling of satisfaction, if not fullness. This sense of satiety is so important to avoid additional craving and hunger that would otherwise tempt you to excessive indulgence and bingeing. If you must cheat, it should be with an occasional treat. You cannot be always chomping at the bit.

Characteristic #6.   Good Digestibility

I'm sure that you have had many a meal preparation that felt good going down, but one or even two hours later, you had serious reservations and regret. Some foods are not easily digested. They are prone to produce any of a wide variety of gastrointestinal upset symptoms. These may include nausea or vomiting, abdominal pain or cramping, diarrhea or constipation, reflux or retching, bilious headache, heartburn, flatulence and more. That's no way to maintain a diet. Food should always be a pleasure, from the first encounter by sight or smell, right down to the last.

The key to good digestion is clearly efficient enzyme action and **The Enzyme Diet**™ takes full account of this and creates a winning difference by including carefully designed and selective digestive enzymes for optimal activity. The result is enhanced digestibility of all foods, a more healthy gastrointestinal mucosa, enhanced nutrient absorption and easier elimination of residual waste.

Characteristic #7.   Personal Flexibility

Of the millions of people across America who can be said to be on a diet today, you can be sure that there is someone of almost every conceivable description. They have different amounts of weight to lose, different expectations, different past experiences and different personal values. Clearly, there is no single diet that will satisfy all their needs or goals. No one size fits all! But the ideal weight loss diet should be flexible enough to allow the vast majority of dieters including you, to take advantage of its benefits for healthy and effective weight reduction.

Some diet plans we found have very strict and limiting specifications. These are in some of the more structured programs where semi-professionals take control of their clients' dietary regimens and impose strict discipline. This might work well for the dieter who is either ill-informed to make their own selections, or is too irresponsible to make the right disciplined choices.

After reading **The Enzyme Diet**™ **Solution** you will be fully equipped to start your own individualized program. You will be able to make appropriate healthy choices on a daily basis that will allow you to lose weight effectively by design and to keep it off.

Characteristic #8.   Lifestyle Change

Clearly, effective weight loss is more than just a diet. It is a lifestyle change. It is more than a quick fix. It means systemic reduction in the short to medium term and effective maintenance in the long run. Although the dietary component is usually the focus in attacking one's weight, and it will again be in this program, it cannot be in isolation.

Even as you limit your intake, your challenge must be faced and fought on at least two other fronts. Physical activity must be increased to essentially burn off existing storage fat and maintain your lean muscle mass. It cannot be overstated that no diet will be adequate in the long run without complementary exercise. Similarly, any attempt to consciously manage your weight must be initiated and pursued with changes in mental attitude and healthy self image to provide all the motivation and self discipline you require to follow through. As such, the ideal weight loss diet will always be a truly comprehensive program that leads to a change of thinking and therefore healthy behavior modification.

The Enzyme Diet™ Solution is a program of self responsibility. It is taking charge of your health and making choices to control your weight through disciplined eating, moderate exercise and positive thinking. It's all there.

Characteristic #9.   Reasonable Affordability

Some diet programs require steep expenditures and we saw earlier that this can be a disincentive to good compliance. But it need not be so. The ideal weight loss diet should essentially only alter your food choices and lead to simple economic substitution that does not call for much additional out of pocket expense.

In fact, your careful dieting might avoid the wasted expenditure on large fattening meals, expensive sweets and treats that you already know are unnecessary and sometimes unhealthy. Fresh, raw natural food alternatives are usually less expensive than the highly processed and preserved fast food selections. Compare the price of a baked potato to all its processed presentations in today's supermarkets and restaurants. Think of the real value of a full course meal and look at the price of a choice meal replacement that delivers all the essential nutrients and without all those empty, fattening calories. **The Enzyme Diet™ Solution** turns out to be a wise, economical and responsible program because it is healthy, effective and definitely affordable.

Characteristic #10.   Essential Safety

Every doctor thinks daily of our Hippocratic oath and the important maxim: *Above all, do no harm.* Whatever else a diet is, it must of necessity be extremely safe. This entire industry has had an unfortunate reputation, in some quarters and at different times, because irresponsible racketeers have exploited the uninformed and desperate weight loss seekers with fad diets that proved disastrous. You've heard of the tragic consequences of some liquid protein diets, for example. Then came a number of herbal preparations with active ingredients that turned out to be stimulants or appetite suppressants which have unhealthy side effects. Then came a succession of diet pills that promised so much and delivered so little beyond clinical illness and morbidity. Fortunately, most of these magic potions are now off the market. The Food and Drug Administration (FDA) has banned over 100 ingredients once found in many over the counter diet products. None of these substances, have proven effective in weight loss or even appetite suppression.

The Enzyme Diet™ therefore includes no caffeine, ephedra or other stimulants and no suspicious herbal ingredients. It is a demonstrably safe and effective method to reduce your caloric intake and to supply all the essential nutrients you need and more, in a simple, affordable and flexible program.

There you have it! The ideal weight loss program will have at least the following ten characteristics just described:

1. **Controlled Calorie**
2. **Adequate Nutrients**
3. **Metabolic Boost**
4. **Enough Variety**
5. **Convenient Satisfaction**
6. **Good Digestibility**
7. **Personal Flexibility**
8. **Lifestyle Change**
9. **Reasonable Affordability**
10. **Essential Safety**

That's the kind of program you should be looking for and that's what you're going to find in **The Enzyme Diet**™ **Solution**. You may have tried another diet and failed because it did not have all ten of these characteristics.

The truth is that to lose weight effectively and to keep it off, nothing but ten-out-of-ten will do. But don't give up, there really is a solution for you.

Now that you know what you're looking for, let's go on to **Part II** to find some real answers to your weight problem, as we explore the details of **The Enzyme Diet**™ **Solution.**

Part II

❧

Your Enzyme Diet
SOLUTION

Are You Forgetting the Missing Link?

❧ *Chapter 4* ❧

THE ESSENCE OF LIFE
A New Awareness

You *should always let the main thing be the main thing.* Whoever first said that cliché, put much profound wisdom into a few simple words. If health is the main thing you could ever possess, what should always be a very high priority in your life? Yes, health comes before weight, before wealth and even before happiness! And when you focus on health at the molecular level, what's really important for getting things done? What makes your cells function? What makes all that intricate metabolism possible? What's the main thing? What comes to your mind?

Just think … it would hardly occur to you otherwise. And the answer is … **Enzymes**!

Of course, you're really not surprised because after all, you're reading **The Enzyme Diet™ Solution.** This is the diet where Enzymes take center stage. They are the real stars of this show and you will see why they would walk away with all the cell's Academy Awards if ever there was such a recognition devised.

In Part 1 of the book, we began by taking a look at the national health and even economic crisis posed by the growing epidemic of overweight and obesity. We made a selective review of the most popular weight loss products and programs that together contribute only an elusive remedy since the overwhelming majority of dieters suffer in frustration from exaggerated expectations and their observed yo-yo dieting experience. We also tried to get a grip on the crux of the problem. We know that it is tempting to blame your genes, your hormones, your environment and anything else that you can think of. But in the final analysis, the evasive search for another culprit leaves you at a loss and you must come back to the basics.

You need to cut back on the amount of energy as food calories that you consume and then unnecessarily store as fat. You need adequate nutrition to feed your cells so you do not starve. You need some way of addressing your metabolic tendency of slowing down to counter your best intentions. You need a comprehensive program that is safe, effective and sustainable. In a word, you need **The Enzyme Diet™ Solution**. That's what we will now elucidate in this second major section. In the final section of the book, we will go into the detailed personal application of the complete program.

But for now, we need to get to know our star players. So it's back to basics, back to school - back to Enzymes 101.

Enzymes 101

Enzymes serve as the body's quiet labor force, participating in every single function required for your daily activities and they truly are indispensable to life itself. They are responsible for executing all the biochemical functions of every organ system in your body. At the same time, they are most important in supporting your body's defenses and immune system to protect you from all the harmful forces and specific dangers to your health. Enzymes process the synthesis of all your DNA and RNA that ultimately control your genetics and define your physical characteristics. They are involved from beginning to end of all healthy activity inside your body.

Dr. Edward Howell was probably the first researcher to emphasize the importance of food enzymes to human nutrition. In 1946, he wrote the book, *"The Status of Food Enzymes in Digestion and Metabolism."* In his own words, ***"Enzymes are substances which make life possible. They are needed for every chemical reaction that occurs in the body. Without enzymes, no activity at all would take place. Neither vitamins, minerals or hormones can do any work without enzymes."***

Dr. Howell announced his discovery of the **Principle of Enzyme Nutrition** even earlier, in 1932. He then devoted the rest of his life, until his death in 1988 (at the age of 93), to researching and teaching about the critical role that enzymes play in nutrition and human health. He published his classic work under the new book title, *Enzyme Nutrition* (Avery, 1985)

Briefly stated, the Principle of Enzyme Nutrition is that **a full complement of digestive enzymes must be ingested along with food for the complete nutritional value of food to be delivered to the cells of the body.** In fact, as we have seen in recent years with the development of a better understanding of the underlying causes of food allergies, incompletely digested food can even become a toxin rather than a nutrient. But ... let's get back to some fundamentals.

WHAT ARE ENZYMES?

Enzymes are proteins. Like all other proteins they consist of long chains of amino acids joined together by the famous linkages called peptide bonds. They are present in all living cells where they control essentially all metabolic processes.

The late Dr. Leo Roy, MD., ND wrote in "*Enzymes - Weavers of Life*" (1997) another interesting definition: "*Enzymes are molecular complexes which perform every biochemical reaction and function in man, animal, plant and nature. They are* **the life of life**."

That last phrase is intriguing and worthy of further reflection. It suggests that there is a secret to life, something behind the scenes that allows the expression of all the vitality and vigor that is associated with all living things. Call it what you will, but conceptually, there is an energy or force, some principle or potential, that maintains life and makes it all happen.

Enzymes are catalysts. Classically, catalysts are defined in high school chemistry as '*substances which promote chemical reactions by which chemicals of one nature are transformed into chemicals of another nature, without the catalytic agent itself being a part of, or being used up in the reaction.*'

But enzymes are also **more than catalysts**. After all, catalysts are only inert substances. Dr. Howell theorized that enzymes '*possess a life energy. For instance, enzymes give off a kind of radiation when they work. This is not true of catalysts. In addition, although enzymes contain proteins - and some contain vitamins - the activity factor in enzymes has never been synthesized.*' His use of the term 'radiation' may be misleading in the twenty first century, with microwave ovens, communication satellites and cellular phones everywhere. But he was pointing to something. This is biology, not chemistry. We're looking at living systems, not just inanimate compounds.

There is still today a philosophy that both the living organism and its enzymes are inhabited by a life energy which is separate and distinct from the caloric energy which is liberated from food by enzyme action. The enzyme complex would thus be defined in biological rather than chemical terms. To put it in a single sentence: '*The enzyme complex* harbors a *protein carrier* inhabited by a *vital energy* factor.' Each of these entities is just as real. You've got to think that through. As a trained chemist, I was puzzled by that paradigm. But as a doctor, I understand the mysteriousness of life. Something beckons at the bedside, beyond the chemicals that keep laboratory technicians busy. '*Tis mystery all.*'

As biological catalysts, it is interesting to note that they perform a function that is completely unique in making life possible in an otherwise inanimate world. We referred in Part 1 to the *First Law of Thermodynamics*. Actually, there are three such classic laws. To put it simply, the Second Law can be stated briefly as *All things spontaneously change in the direction of increasing disorder or chaos*. Look around you and you will notice, everything is going downhill. Water evaporates, dust accumulates, salt dissolves in water, papers get scattered, etc., etc. Everything tends to more confusion and lower energy.

But there is one notable exception. **Life!** The process of life is to take a few pounds of earth and lots of water and oxygen, and to organize that insignificant collection of matter into a living, breathing, thinking, reproducing human being. From the simplest unicellular forms of life to the most complex brains, the direction of life is against the grain of everything else in our environment. We thrive at the expense of the environment. Perhaps the biggest clue to why this all happens is that enzymes make the improbable, probable. They cause unlikely change to become realistic. They make inefficient processes virtually 100% efficient. They allow life to happen. *They are indeed the life of life!*

The secrets to enzyme activity, although they really are not secrets anymore, lie in the structure or shape of these large molecules, and secondly, in the positive or negative local charges associated with their individual atoms surrounding reaction sites. Forgive me if I seem fascinated by this, but it is one of the best wonders of nature. The structure of each enzyme is on four levels. First, there is the sequence of amino acids as they are linked together to make a chain, based on the genetic code of corresponding DNA. One wrong substitution can give rise to diseases like sickle cell anemia.

On the second level, the enzyme amino acid sequence gives each one a characteristic coiling pattern - typically a kind of helix with kinks and twists, if you like. Then at the third level, the coils fold or wrap in such a way as to create pockets or nesting places for the reacting molecules to interact - a platform for their union. Finally, some enzymes like hemoglobin consist of more than one chain and these agglomerate (or simply come together and associate) in specific spatial orientations to create unique three-dimensional structures for the reactions to take place. But in all this arrangement, the specificity is paramount. Each enzyme is designed for a particular type of bond cleavage or synthesis. What phenomenal design!

The net efficiency is so good that the reaction rates are astronomical compared to how you or I would do anything. One molecule of an enzyme like catalase for example, found copiously in the liver or in red blood cells, can in one minute break down 5,000,000 molecules of hydrogen peroxide into water and oxygen. All that happens at one active reaction site, one molecule at a time! What an incredible technology!!

Dr. Howell later advanced the elaborate *Food Enzyme Concept* which holds that **organisms endow enzymes with a vital activity factor that is exhaustible**. The capacity of a living organism to make enzymes he called the **Enzyme Potential**. It is consumable and limited. Again, that is all biology. It is a life model, not a ball-and-stick caricature.

I recall what I first learned in high school about electrons. In the Bohr atom, they were particles. That gave me a conceptual idea - a model. It accounted for electron properties and behavior. Later, I learned electrons were waves. That made me think differently. A shift in paradigm. The wave could now explain diffraction patterns and much, much more. But whatever became of the particle? Now, we're not sure. Add to that the evolution of 21st century quantum physics and I don't know how to think. Waves, particles ... trying to put it all together, I'm confused. Scientists refer to that as the duality of nature. It's really double-talk. But electrons are just as real. They are whatever they are, no matter what scientists think of them. And each idea only gives us new insight.

Let's apply the same 'duality of nature' idea to enzymes and recognize them both chemically and biologically. Enzymes do indeed represent the *life element* which is biologically recognized and which can be measured in terms of enzyme activity. Perhaps the easiest way to recognize this is to note when chemical reactions fail to occur because enzymes are not present, e.g. when a radiated or cooked potato fails to sprout. In that case, the life element of the food enzymes is destroyed by radiation or heat, even if no real chemical bonds are broken.

So, for the purpose of our presentation of enzymes, let us consider that the proteins in enzymes serve merely as carriers of enzyme activity factors. We can therefore summarize that **enzymes are protein carriers charged biologically with vital energy factors**, just as your car battery consists of metal plates charged with electrical energy.

That is a very useful paradigm or model. You may need to make a paradigm shift. And that's okay. It makes for a new understanding and opens up practical innovation as we explore the general area of enzyme nutrition.

WHAT ROLES DO ENZYMES PLAY?

Just to illustrate how diverse this vital energy factor must be, let's reflect on some of the biological roles they are called on to perform. Enzymes control or carry out every function by which our bodies :

- Utilize food and energy;
- Develop new structures;
- Act and react;
- Maintain health;
- Heal injury;
- Restore wellness;
- Protect from all threats;
- Detoxify themselves.

And that's just to mention a few broad classes of activity. If we were to consider the individual physiological processes taking place continuously in the body, we might then recognize that enzymes activate :

- Every brain impulse by which we think;
- Every muscle contraction by which we move;
- Every nerve signal by which we feel;
- Every hormone by which cells communicate;
- Every chemical change by which we digest and assimilate foods;
- Every process to neutralize toxins or discard dead cells;
- Every event of cell division and growth;
- Every other conceivable function and expression of living.

There is hardly any other comparable molecular performer or process in the body. Enzymes are ubiquitous but nothing could be more targeted for rapid, specific and critical action. In real terms, each enzyme has but one, and only one, very specific action. It has an affinity for, and a control over, a specific type of chemical bond. Every molecule of every substance is bound to other molecules by such bonds. The bonds which hold molecules together are specific to those molecules and each enzyme acts on one specific type of bond.

All enzymes act in one of two different ways. They tend to either **break the bonds** and split apart molecules, or they can **create the bonds** which hold molecules together. These simple changes combine to define life by a process that is generally called metabolism. Enzymes are therefore the key - the neglected secret of life itself.

Enzymes create the difference between live and dead cells. If cells cannot manufacture and utilize all their enzymes, there can be no normal structures or functions of those cells. How much more critical could anything get?

Even the nature of cells depends on the types and organization of specific enzyme groups. As we mentioned, DNA is synthesized by enzymes. One type of DNA and its genes write the code for the enzymes that create say, liver cells, whereas other types create other types of cells, organs and tissues. Changes in cell structure can be caused by changes in enzymes or enzymatic activity. **All biochemical activities inside cells are orchestrated by enzymes**. Some act upon and affect proteins. Others act on our genes and their nucleic acid and DNA components.

The main organ of enzyme activities is the liver. Our livers are like tiny complex laboratories working with hundreds of thousands of enzyme technicians. These perform biochemical tasks which would require a fully equipped, completely staffed laboratory perhaps the size of a major city. Our blood carries every toxin, body waste, poison and carcinogen, into our livers. These are neutralized and destroyed there by our liver enzymes. The liver converts these toxins and other products into molecular forms that can be readily handled, flushed out and eliminated.

Enzymes are our white blood cell's poison-destroying agents. They digest their targets in ways identical to the enzymes produced by the pancreas. They destroy (digest) blood toxins and disease-producing substances, blood clots, cholesterol and other substances that deposit on blood vessel walls and create blockages. They detoxify the substances which nourish or poison bacteria and viruses. They help counteract inflammation, infections and fevers. They relieve pain. **They provide these benefits in ways much more effectively than drugs or other treatments**. And they do that all so naturally!

Food and other substances consisting of multiple complexes of molecules undergo multiple changes -- one modification of their chemical structure at a time. One enzyme works on a substance at one stage - then another enzyme takes over and produces the next change - then another and another. They work in cascades, until finally the changes required to create a specific end substance are complete. All this proceeds at tremendous speeds. According to Dr. Leo Roy, one of the fastest enzymes, called carboanhydrase, changes up to 36 million target molecules in one minute. That's simply amazing. It's incomprehensible!

Clearly, you must be getting the message. Enzymes are everywhere in the body, facilitating if not controlling life itself. *The life of life* is a great definition. But when was the last time you thought about your enzymes? You hear every day about vitamins. You probably worry about your cholesterol. But what about your enzymes? Do you ever give attention to them? You owe your life to them. But like others, you probably just take them for granted.

It never ceases to amaze me how presumptuous we are. When things are going well, we could hardly care less. But when something goes wrong, then we focus. As a doctor, this pardigm is so common in the office, the emergency room or in the home, where patients experience all kinds of trouble through neglect.

Just like that, I wonder why enzymes get so little press.

HOW TO CLASSIFY ENZYMES?

There are three broad classes of enzymes:
  1. **Digestive enzymes**, which digest our food;
  2. **Metabolic enzymes**, which run our bodies;
  3. **Food enzymes** from raw foods, which start food digestion.

Digestive Enzymes:

No matter what we eat - whether it is grilled, baked, fried, canned, steamed, whatever - we consume essentially three basic bulk food materials: proteins, carbohydrates and fats. In order to convert these large complex macromolecules into smaller and simpler biochemical substances that we can use, we need specific groups of enzymes. These are the enzymes secreted principally by organs of the gastrointestinal system including the salivary glands, stomach, pancreas and intestines. These organs produce groups of enzymes which are each conditioned for the different environments at each stage along the digestive tract: These are summarized in **Table 4:**

Table 4	**Digestive Enzymes**
• *Amylases* in the saliva:	These start the digestion of sugars and starches even before they reach the stomach.
• *Pepsins* in the stomach:	These split some peptide bonds which hold all protein molecules together.
• *Proteases* and *peptidases* of the pancreas:	These complete protein digestion.
• *Lipases* of the pancreas:	These digest fats and oils.
• *Amylases* of the pancreas:	These complete the digestion of sugars and starches in the intestines.

Enzyme digestion is the process that our bodies use to obtain the nutrients they need to nourish cells, to maintain health and to create cell structures and functions. No nutrient becomes available to or utilizable by cells unless there is a transformation by the action of enzymes. They break down the large food molecules so that they are small enough to pass into the blood through the minute channels of the intestines and are in chemical forms acceptable to, and utilizable by cells and tissues.

Digestive enzymes are powerful agents but they do not digest the body's own proteins - fortunately so. In health, all the cells of the stomach and intestines and all body cells in general, are "untouchables" - at least until they have reached the end of their life span, or have dangerously mutated, or have become denatured in some way. Then the digestive enzymes will attack and digest all those cells that are worn out or dying, as well as those that are foreign or abnormal. Unfortunately, in patients with inflammatory bowel disease, the cell lining or mucosa does become vulnerable and there are clinical consequences.

Chemicals and abnormal toxic substances may demolish enzymes - but foods do not. Have you ever wondered what happens to your enzymes that are secreted to digest your food? Once their task in the intestines has been accomplished, the digestive enzymes do not disappear. They are far too precious! They mix in with the foods and accompany them as they filter through the intestinal walls. They are carried through the gut wall and then released. Passing into our bodies, they are in no way hampered. They are not bound to specific receptors or taken up by "roaming" lymphocytes as though they were foreign intruders. They are naturally-occurring proteins. In the blood stream they are bound to carriers which protect and block them from destruction.

Throughout our bodies the digestive enzymes actually perform a scavenging and "house cleaning" role. They help to decompose whatever dead cells they contact. They handle foreign substances anywhere throughout our bodies as effectively as they digest foods in the intestines. They digest the cell debris which comprise the leftovers of cell breakdown as well as all toxic body wastes. They digest toxic bacteria, viruses and fungi, parasites, worms and amoebae. These too, like foods, are made up of proteins and minerals. But they have chemical "fingerprints" which are different from body cells. This leaves them vulnerable to enzymes.

The marvelous powers that our digestive enzymes have for processing foods could leave us with the impression that they are all powerful. Such is not the case. Their digestive powers are limited. Without the help of other enzymes, they cannot process *all* the cell or food components. They need to work in conjunction with enzymes secreted by the cells themselves.

Of course, in the context of weight loss, we are particularly interested in the enzymes that digest fat. These are the *lipases* produced for food digestion in the gut and for later action after they are absorbed. Lipases are also produced by fat cells themselves. They are assigned the role of fat consumption, if you like. They act when released at the appropriate time to discard stored fat and/or to release the energy required from this reserve.

Stored in organelles called "lysozomes", in every cell, are different kinds of special enzymes. When cells are worn out or used up (in other words, their life cycle is finished), or if cells are damaged, the membranes of these lysozomes rupture and release their enzymes. These cell enzymes auto-digest the cells' components in preparation for elimination. They bring about the eventual compost and return to the soil, of all discarded organic matter.

Metabolic Enzymes

All our cells, organs and tissues are run by metabolic enzymes. These enzyme workers take the amino acids, free fatty acids and sugars from the digestion of proteins, fats and carbohydrates, and structure them with water, oxygen and a few lesser players, into healthy, properly working bodies. Just think how amazing that really is! All the technology known to man that has brought about our modern civilization is but a very simple exercise, in comparison to the myriad of complex diversities being executed constantly inside our cells. Every organ and tissue has its own particular metabolic enzymes to do specialized work. They take the same basic ingredients and assemble them with precision into vastly different products that all function together in near perfect harmony. Think of your beating heart or your thinking brain or just your blinking eye. A final product of soil, air and water. Enzymes at work! Incredible, but true!

Modern research is implicating enzymes in all our activities. Even abstract thinking involves some enzyme activity. In 1930, 80 enzymes were known; in 1947, 200; in 1957, 660; in 1962, 850 and by 1968, scientists had identified 1300 of them. Today more than 5,000 metabolic enzymes have been identified that run the body chemistry and are involved in all body processes including breathing, talking, movement, behavior and maintaining the immune system, among other things. Although thousands of enzymes are known, many more reactions have been identified, for which the particular enzymes responsible are not yet known. Thousands of metabolic enzymes are necessary to carry on the work of the body, to repair damage and decay, and to heal in disease states. They were appropriately described earlier as carrying on *the life of life*.

Since good health depends on all these thousands of metabolic enzymes doing an excellent job, we must be sure that nothing interferes with the body making enough of them. A shortage could cause serious trouble, very serious indeed. Now keep that thought in mind.

Food Enzymes

All uncooked foods contain an abundance of food enzymes which correspond to the type of nutrients they provide. Those foods with relatively high fat content like dairy, oils, seeds and nuts, contain higher concentrations of the fat digesting enzyme lipase. Grains which provide carbohydrates also contain higher concentrations of amylase and less lipase or proteases. Lean meats, on the other hand, are a good source of protein and they have the protease in the form of cathepsin and little amylase. Even low calorie foods like fruits and vegetables have mainly the important cellulase enzymes to help break down the plant fibers.

The question arises: Why? Why do these particular enzymes exist in the appropriate foods? The answer is compelling. These enzymes in food help to pre-digest these foods upon human consumption. They spare the body the extra burden of secreting more enzymes for complete digestion.

Plants grown on healthy, mineral-rich and balanced soils, absorb the elements they require to make generous amounts of enzymes. They create enzymes, but it is only in the process of, and at the stage of ripening of foods, that they complete the creation of their enzymes and vitamins. Again, the question arises: Why? To fulfil their destiny? Picked ripe and eaten while still fresh, such foods provide us with rich nutrients and enzymes most essential to our health and healing.

Bananas will illustrate this point very well. Green bananas have about 20% starch. As they ripen, the enzyme amylase breaks down the starch and each banana changes to 20% sugar. About one quarter of this sugar is dextrose (similar to glucose) and needs no further digestion. Ripe bananas would hardly make you fat. Incidentally, the same enzymes in bananas have little or no effect on other starches like potato starch, for example.

All enzyme systems need to be constantly replaced or replenished. This is done best by eating live, fresh, healthy, chemical-free, undercooked, natural foods and herbs, grown on healthy, mineral-rich soils and preserved in this state as they are taken into our bodies as foods. Herbs refer to those plants which have absorbed trace minerals or synthesized bioactive molecules that are specially implicated for healing specific ailments.

Any kind of **heat treatment of food** in the kitchen **destroys enzymes**. Slow or fast baking, slow or fast boiling, stewing and frying all destroy up to 100 percent of the enzymes in food. Most enzymes are denatured above a temperature of about 118 degrees F. Vigorous boiling takes place at 212 degrees F. Frying is done at a much higher temperature, and in addition to destroying enzymes, it also damages protein, or forms new chemical compounds with unknown and possibly pathogenic possibilities, imposing still more burden upon the metabolic enzymes. Although baking takes place at 300° to 400° F, it is in dry heat, so the effect is no more destructive than at boiling temperatures. Enzymes are completely destroyed at all these temperatures!

Enzymes are also destroyed by exposure to oxygen or to radiation and a host of commercial processes used in the food industry. The food may look the same and even taste the same, but it could be as different as chalk from cheese, one with no enzymes and therefore no life, in contrast to the live, enzyme-rich composition of healthy food.

There is no substitute for food enzymes. That's why we pointed out that in fact, there is only one enzyme factory on the face of the earth: the living cell. **Only Nature knows how to manufacture food enzymes.** No chemist or drug company or laboratory can. We only *harvest* nature's product. We can and do synthesize digestive aids but do not confuse antacids and motility agents with enzymes.

Nature's plan seems to call for *food enzymes* to help with digestion instead of forcing the body's digestive enzymes to carry the whole load. If food enzymes do some of the work, the enzyme potential can allot less activity to digestive enzymes, and have much more to give to the hundreds of metabolic enzymes that run the entire body.

Yes, if food enzymes did some of the work, the enzyme potential of normal people would probably not be facing impending bankruptcy, as it is now in the bodies of millions of people who survive on the 'minus diet' - a diet of food *minus its natural enzymes.* Their enzyme potential has a problem somewhat similar to an NSF checking account which tends to become dangerously deficient if not continually replenished.

The practice of dietary supplementation is a wise contemporary solution to replace vital nutrients and other factors that should be present in the diets but which have been removed, destroyed or simply neglected. That includes enzymes. Perhaps you've never thought of it, but now you know the value.

Taking digestive enzymes in a supplement form may prove to be essential to your health. There are no hazards or threats to your well being in using them, or even using them in significant amounts. In this way, you can add or make deposits to that same checking account in the analogy above. You will then be truly rich!

The Food Enzyme Concept

The Food Enzyme Concept was the subtitle of the book *Enzyme Nutrition* (Avery, 1985) by Dr. Edward Howell. It more or less summarizes his life's work. This concept of Dr. Howell introduces a different way of looking at nutrition in health and disease. It heralds a revolution in our understanding of disease processes.

According to this novel concept, enzymes possess biological, as well as chemical, properties. When you ingest them, the enzymes in raw food, (as well as supplementary enzymes), result in a significant degree of digestion, thus lowering the drain on your own enzyme potential. But remember that these are statements of biology, not chemistry. It is a way of thinking that gives new insights into how and why the body functions as it does.

Although your body makes less than two dozen digestive enzymes, it probably uses up more of your enzyme potential to supply these *in bulk*, compared to what it uses to make the thousands of *trace* metabolic enzymes needed to keep all your organs and tissues functioning with their diversified activities.

This Food Enzyme Concept has significant practical implications in today's world. To fully grasp its meaning, we must explain five basic insights that it provides.

Insight #1 - The Law of Adaptive Secretion of Digestive Enzymes

If the human organism must devote a huge portion of its enzyme potential to making digestive enzymes, that spells trouble for the whole body. There is a strain on production of metabolic enzymes because of this and there may not be enough enzyme potential to go around. In other words, there is a perceived competition for production between the two classes of enzymes.

In 1943, the physiology laboratory of Northwestern University established the *Law of Adaptive Secretion of Digestive Enzymes* by experiments on rats [1]. The amount of digestive enzymes secreted by the pancreas in response to carbohydrate, protein and fat was measured and it was found that the concentration of each enzyme varied with the amount of each of these food materials it was called upon to digest.

The Law of Adaptive Secretion of Digestive Enzymes holds that *the organism values its enzymes so highly that it will make no more than is needed for the job.* If some of the food is digested by enzymes available in the food, the body will need to make less concentrated enzymes. This Law has since been confirmed by dozens of university laboratories throughout the world.

Insight #2 - The Food-Enzyme Stomach - Food Enzyme Digestion in Humans

According to the Food Enzyme Concept, there is a mechanism operating in all creatures permitting food enzymes to digest a particular fraction of the food in which they are contained. In humans, the upper portion of the stomach is in fact a food-enzyme stomach. This part secretes no enzymes. It behaves the same as other food-enzyme stomachs. When raw food is eaten, it goes into this peristalis-free, food-enzyme section of the stomach where these food enzymes begin to digest the food.

In fact, the digestion of the protein, carbohydrate and fat in raw food begins in the mouth at the very moment the plant cell walls are ruptured, releasing the food enzymes during the act of mastication. After swallowing, digestion continues in the food-enzyme section of the stomach for about 30 minutes to an hour, or until the rising tide of acidity reaches a point where it is inhibited. Then the stomach enzyme, pepsin, takes over.

If the food is cooked, the naturally occurring enzymes are destroyed and what you then have is essentially enzyme-free foods. When this is swallowed, it settles in a mass in the same food-enzyme section of the stomach, where it waits for the same period of up to 30 minutes to an hour. During this time, nothing much happens to it. If harmful bacteria are swallowed with the food, they may attack it during this time of enforced idleness. The salivary enzyme works on the carbohydrate, but the protein and fat must wait.

This is where proper digestive enzyme supplements fit in. Taken with the meal, these exogenous digestive enzymes begin immediate digestion of all nutrients. Whatever digestion is accomplished by enzyme supplements or food enzymes, does not have to be done by the digestive enzymes of the body. Eating raw or unprocessed foods or adding enzyme supplements with meals therefore allows the body to devote its attention to supplying more metabolic enzymes for use by the organs and tissues to carry on their functions, provide repairs and bring about cures.

Now let's put these two key ideas together to derive an important conclusion.

The discovery of the *Food-Enzyme Stomach* and the discovery of the *Law of Adaptive Secretion of Digestive Enzymes* are keys to the Food Enzyme Concept. If your stomach is performing its proper role and you are eating much of your foods uncooked, a large portion of your intake will be partially digested before reacting with the stronger digestive juices found there.

Moreover, if you eat uncooked food, or if you use whole food preparations containing complementary enzymes, fewer of your body's internal digestive enzymes will be called upon to perform the digestive function. That is, your body adapts to the plentiful supply of enzymes in the uncooked foods or supplements, by secreting less of its own digestive enzymes - this preserves your internal enzyme supplies for the important work of maintaining metabolic harmony!

But if your foods are all cooked and the enzymes destroyed, then enzymes must be supplemented to preserve your body's production of enzymes in accordance with the Law of Adaptive Secretion.

If you are a sports fan, you can think of it in this way. Metabolic enzymes and digestive enzymes are like two teams, A and B. The metabolic enzymes would have to be the A-Team because the body places a higher and more selective or specialized function on these more limited metabolic enzymes. They are the critical players controlling all cellular metabolism and activity. When the B-Team does not show up for their games or has a number of players on the injured list, then A-players are summoned to substitute in the B-games and are then not available for their own critical A-games. Then you lose the prized trophies. It is a waste of potential and skills for any good manager to deploy his key major league players to substitute in the minor leagues. Nature is far too wise for that. That's why enzymes are supplied in raw, wholesome natural foods. They stack up the B-team roster with lots of extras, to preserve the best players on the A team.

Did that help you, sports fans? If you make sure that you have an adequate supply of digestive enzymes (and that really means enough food enzymes or supplementary enzymes), then you spare your metabolic enzymes and preserve them in good form for their most important duties.

In the context of weight loss, with **The Enzyme Diet™**, there is more reserve potential for maintaining your metabolic rate and for making lipase in your fat cells - that's the enzyme you recall, that digests stored fat to get it moving.

That's a major key right there. We saw in Part I the big challenge of maintaining metabolic rate during any attempt at weight loss. Now we have at least one innovative idea: **it is possible to indirectly affect metabolic rate by preserving the enzyme potential with the judicious use of supplementary enzymes.**

Pause. Don't rush past that conclusion. It is an idea worth pondering. It's neither intuitive nor instinctive, but it is very insightful. It's another paradigm shift. It's a way of understanding nutrition that you've probably never considered. It's not on nutrition labels or even in dietary textbooks, but it is critical for effective weight loss, as we will see in detail later. So before you move on, just take another moment to reflect on what you just learned.

Go ahead and think. Think about that! But think outside the box! Think until the light dawns.

Insight #3 - Enzyme Wastage

We are guilty of being careless about our enzymes. They are among the most precious assets we possess and we should welcome outside enzyme help. If we depend solely upon the potential enzymes we inherit, they will be used up just like inherited money that is not supplemented by a steady income. The Food Enzyme Concept points out that acute wastage of large quantities of enzymes is strenuously objected to by the body.

In an experiment in 1944, young rats and chickens were fed a diet of raw soybeans (high in enzyme inhibitors) and huge quantities of pancreatic digestive enzymes were wasted in combating the inhibitors. The pancreas gland enlarged to handle the extra burden, and the animals became sick and failed to grow [2]. Those early experiments proved that organisms tend to rebel against having their enzymes wasted. They have now been repeated and amplified in dozens of scientific experimental laboratories.

We are guilty of forcing our precious enzyme activity to do all the menial work of digestion and then expect it to also do a perfect job with metabolism. Food enzymes and other exogenous enzymes can help with digestion, but not with metabolism. Then why not let these helper-enzymes free the body's energy stores to more efficiently run the metabolism of the body? That makes consummate sense.

Insight #4 - Fixed Enzyme Potential or Enzyme Bank Account

In his book, *Enzyme Nutrition - The Food Enzyme Concept* (1985), Dr. Howell presented evidence that clearly indicates the existence of a fixed enzyme potential in all living creatures. This potential diminishes in time, subject to the conditions and pace of life.

Humans eating an enzymeless diet, use up a tremendous amount of their enzyme potential in lavish secretions of the pancreas and other digestive organs. The result is a shortened lifespan, illness and lowered resistance to stresses of all types, psychological and environmental. On the other hand, by eating foods with their enzymes intact and by supplementing cooked foods with additional enzymes, we can in principle stop many abnormal and pathological aging processes. As a consequence of the improvements in health on such a regime, symptoms are alleviated and the response of the body's immune system is strengthened.

Let's put it another way, as in our earlier analogy. The more you take out of the enzyme potential bank, the less you will have in it, until finally you have more blank checks at the end than cash in the bank. Most people spend their enzyme bank account and seldom make a deposit. Since various experiments have taught us that enzymes are precious commodities, it would be wiser to conserve enzymes and get enzyme reinforcements from the outside. It should not be hard to see how the enzyme bank account of the body can get out of balance through heavy withdrawals and skimpy deposits. In a different metaphor, perhaps we could conclude that life naturally ends when our enzymes get tired and these overburdened workers collapse or just throw in the towel.

Orthodox chemistry likes to maintain that the harmful effect heat has on enzymes is due to denaturization of their protein. But it shies away from the biological responses to temperature changes. It cannot explain why enzymes work harder in a test tube at 80° F than at 40° F, and die sooner at the higher temperature.   In both instances the same enzyme mechanism operates and it imparts new meaning to the contention that life is an enzyme process, ending when the enzyme potential becomes depleted beyond a certain point. That too requires some biological thinking outside the box.

Insight #5 - Absorption of Enzymes

It is widely assumed that enzymes cannot be absorbed into the organism because they are a protein-based molecule, too large to pass through the intestinal mucosa. This view is theoretical, originating in the chemical laboratory after futile attempts to make unsplit proteins pass through inert, nonliving membranes.

Experience has shown that this matter requires the use of biological, not chemical, laboratories. Biological research requires more time and effort. Aside from this, researchers have pointed out that some molecules smaller than enzymes are not absorbed, while ferritin, with a molecular weight of 500,000, is absorbed [3]. They suggested that absorption was governed by factors other than molecular size.

To put the question of enzyme absorption into sharp focus, research has shown that when only a fraction of the total volume of digestive enzymes secreted into the gastrointestinal canal is lost to the living organism, death results in less than a week [4]. Does not this alone prove that the tremendous biological value of the total digestive enzyme secretions, including the saliva, gastric juice and pancreatic juice, must be reabsorbed into the organism as a normal, physiological daily event?

Enzymes are something more than ordinary proteins - they are a corollary of life. Further, the fact that the living organism strongly rebels when it is forced to waste even a small fraction of its enzymes every day, again confirms that the absorption of enzymes through the wall of the intestine is an indispensable and daily physiological act.

Numerous studies have confirmed that enzymes are absorbed in the intestinal tract. Many whole proteins, including plant and animal enzymes, have been shown in human and animal studies to be absorbed intact into the bloodstream following oral administration. We will come back to this shortly.

However, before we discuss putting enzymes to work, let's first set the stage by defining some boundaries between nutrition and medicine. This important interface between nutrition and medicine has been blurred so much and for so long that it has grossly impeded the path to better health and wellness.

Nutrition And Medicine

It is always a mistake whenever one approaches the whole area of nutrition in the typical mindset of the doctor and the use of pharmaceutical drugs. This is so common, but it leads to totally wrong conclusions and applications.

The medical model is fundamentally designed around diagnosis and cure. It is after the fact. If you have a clinical problem, the doctor first wants to find a diagnosis. We label the condition. Then we use our encyclopedia of cumulative knowledge to scan all the therapies known, to carefully select the best therapeutic drug or other therapy to prescribe, and when indicated, the best surgical procedure to perform. This is heroic medicine at its best. Intervening to kill pain, to stop bleeding, to resuscitate the heart, to remove whatever ails the patient - that's the approach of acute allopathic medicine, and it should be. There is no substitute for acute care. That's why doctors exist - to counteract disease and to save lives!

Acute care is focused and goal oriented. It is specific in application. Whatever the doctor does is targeted at a specific organ or cell type or microorganism. You must take *this* (pill, therapy or surgery), because you have *that* (symptom, diagnosis or disease). Most such interventions are also unnatural. We use foreign substances that are unknown to the body in its normal function. We trick or fool the body in some way to force it to act or react differently. Most of the time, this is beneficial and often curative. Sometimes we have to live with the undesirable consequences. We call those necessary side effects and complications. So the doctor is always doing risk-benefit analysis with the Hippocratic oath ever in mind - '*above all, do no harm.*'

Nutrition is an entirely different matter. This is a *universal, indispensable and daily activity.* We all eat to feed our bodies because they are designed to utilize essential nutrients continuously. Feeding the body is not a reaction to anything. We eat even when we are most healthy and have absolutely no complaint but our natural instinct. We have internal systems in our brain that stimulate our hunger as the natural drive to preserve life. Appetite is a life saving gift. Loss of appetite is clinically symptomatic.

Nutrition then, is first *preventative in nature.* It is not necessarily curative and needs no preliminary diagnosis. One need not ever justify eating. It is always normal, natural and necessary to consume all the essential nutrients. These are the vital ingredients of the proven foods that we choose to eat. We never need to do a history and physical or even worse, undergo a batch of laboratory tests and procedures to justify a daily diet. Neither do we need to wait until we observe the consequences of nutritional deficiency. There need not be any symptom, diagnosis or disease to prompt action. Only life! **We eat to live, not to cure! Diet is primarily defensive!**

The classic diseases like scurvy, pellagra, rickets and all the other medically recognized deficiency conditions are mostly a thing of the past, at least in contemporary, industrialized societies. Those are not the issues of nutrition today. Rather, we are compelled to think of the leading causes of widespread degenerative diseases, most of which are known to have a strong association with cumulative dietary habits. No one would deny today the role of nutrition in cardiovascular disease, including heart disease and stroke, or in cancer, in most gastrointestinal illnesses, in osteoporosis, in diabetes, hypertension, kidney disease and a host of other chronic degenerative conditions. In fact, nutrition today is as important in health as in disease. Again, the role of nutrition is primarily preventative and not necessarily curative. That alone negates the application of the usual medical model here.

Most of the time, nutritional intervention is *taken for granted*. It is not newsworthy. There are no heroes. You do what's good for you - you eat - and that's that. If you benefit from eating lots of fresh fruits and raw vegetables, for example, don't expect anyone to applaud or request an interview. You're just doing the natural, healthy thing. So what's the big deal? There's no reason for a heroic drama series on television to show how ordinary folk change the quality and quantity of their lives by eating right.

Nutrition is also *non-specific*. Just think of this. When you had your last meal, you had no immediate intentions for any of the foods you ate. You simply consumed your full course breakfast, lunch or dinner and forgot it. Your body did everything else. Somehow, your food was absorbed and distributed throughout the body and every cell that needed nutrients went fishing in your blood stream to find what it needed. No one knows exactly what any given cell needs at any given moment. But each cell does. The most fundamental concept of nutrition ought to be summarized in three simple words:

CELLS SELF-SERVE!

The role of nutrition is to provide the complete smorgasbord of nutrients to the body but after that, the cells are on their own. Each one for itself. That is in part, the essence of life. Cells discriminate in their own self interest. We are all humbled by their unimaginable wisdom and discretion. We observe in awe for they are the heroes in the arena of nutrition, not the professionals in white coats.

We teach our cells nothing. When science advances, we unlock the secret of nature so we can better alter the side show. But the central drama of life continues spontaneously, essentially unaffected by our relatively simplistic interventions. We learn surgical technique but only the living body can join the skin in apposition to allow us to remove the sutures. We stop the heart to perform sophisticated and difficult cardiac surgery, but after all our best efforts, when the button is pushed to restart the heart, we hold our breath in tenuous anticipation of the miracle of the next heart beat that negates or affirms whatever changes were done. The point is that life is autonomous and spontaneous. We breathe and feed and life happens. But we must breathe and we must feed. That's life!

Nutrition is a *natural activity*. The foods we eat are the very essentials of life. The body is designed for those nutrients and the nutrients for the body. Real food is typically harmless and safe - at least, in moderation. That's why we seldom think of side effects and complications like we have to always consider with therapeutic drugs. Food is the normal response to simply living. We're all in it together. What a contrast to medicine which has to be carefully individualized and cautiously justified only when absolutely indicated.

So what are enzymes? Are they foods or drugs? The answer is obvious. Enzymes are naturally occurring proteins found in the very type of foods we all eat everyday. They are nothing but sophisticated and complex arrangements of the same 22 essential amino acids that constitute all the body proteins. They exist in food as the essential work force of the plant and animal cells we consume. But they exist for our benefit. They serve the body's needs in aiding digestion, transport and metabolism. They need no justification other than their inescapable presence in the foods we eat. **Enzymes clearly belong in the nutritional domain and not in the medical model.** As such, they ought to be considered as natural ingredients designed for preserving health. They need not be used only for specific intervention as drugs, and one need not be anxious about side effects and complications. One needs no license for their use, since their benefit to risk ratio is as high as the foods we eat.

Unfortunately, we destroy the enzymes in foods by cooking, baking, radiation and commercial processing. Raw foods are rich in enzymes but when we process them, we deplete this valuable gift and put an unnecessary burden on our bodies to cope with what's left behind for consumption. Amazing, isn't it?

Now we can think of putting enzymes to work. That's a nutritional intervention that should find universal application. And that includes you.

࿊

Putting Enzymes To Work

You can put enzymes to work for you. First, by increasing your consumption of raw foods. Fresh fruits and raw vegetables are the obvious starting point. Then consider raw honey; germinated, inhibitor-free, raw cereal grains and seeds; and germinated, inhibitor-free raw nuts. Raw fish like the Japanese love, and careful selection of good certified unpasteurized milk and dairy products, where available, are next in line. Then, when food selection is made, always opt for the least processed and lightly cooked alternatives. After all this, supplementary enzymes, especially plant enzymes, make good sense as part of a complete healthy nutrition plan. Just like vitamins and minerals, they ought not to be taken for granted. Long before clinical therapy is indicated, enzymes are justified as an essential ingredient of nutritional insurance, substituting for what should be always present in our daily intake but what could be lacking for any number of reasons.

It is estimated that some 40% of Americans or more use nutritional supplements on a regular basis. Of course, vitamins top the list. Yet it is interesting to observe that **the main function of vitamins in the body is to support the activity of enzymes**. Vitamins are the supporting cast and enzymes are really the lead actors in the metabolic drama. But we've focused the spotlight for the major part of the last century on vitamins and neglected the central role of enzymes.

These naturally occurring bioactive proteins are known to perform specific roles but that is just the beginning. Our cells know far better what they do. Our role is again to ingest the food enzymes provided by nature and let all the benefits follow.

What are some of the specifics that we already know? Clearly, digestion is the place to begin.

i) Digestive Enzymes for your gut

Lactose intolerance is the classic clinically recognized condition in this area. Lactose is a low molecular weight carbohydrate (a disaccharide milk sugar) that is present in milk and dairy products. It is broken down in the intestines by the action of an enzyme called lactase (enzymes usually end in-ase) into galactose and glucose which are then absorbed. Lactase is generally present in the gut in early childhood and then declines with age. By age 4 or 5, most of the world's population is no longer equipped to handle lactose in the diet. There is a clear genetic predisposition to this lactose intolerance: Blacks have up to 90%, Caucasians about 20-40%, and Orientals somewhere in the middle.

When the enzyme is not effective, lactose remains in the gut to be broken down by bacterial fermentation, producing acids, carbon dioxide and hydrogen gas. These lead to the common symptoms associated with lactose intolerance: diarrhea, gas and abdominal cramps. So what to do if you suffer from lactose intolerance? There is now a commercial source of the lactase enzyme called Lactaid™, available as tablets or drops. Lactese™ is a special milk, made available with low lactose content, for those who wish to drink milk despite their lactose intolerance. Of course, lactose-free soya milk is a simple, natural alternative in this regard.

All foods are naturally rich in different nutrients, including enzymes. All foods need to be digested as a preparation for absorption. When indigestion takes place, a wide variety of symptoms can occur and the cells ultimately lose out because of inadequate absorption. Gastroenterologists deal with the symptoms of incomplete digestion everyday. Many patients present with abdominal cramps, pain, flatulence, malodorous (foul) stools, diarrhea, bloating, nausea, vomiting, rumbling - any of these could be a symptom of incomplete digestion.

But that's all after the fact. One need not experience malabsorption syndrome or gastro-intestinal upset to justify the use of digestive enzymes. As we said before, they are a normal, natural and necessary part of dietary intake. You can add enzymes to your dietary intake *just because they ought to be there.* Many symptoms seem to be alleviated by this simple intervention.

Another example might be that of **celiac disease** (sprue). This is a disease also associated with inadequate digestion but clinically understood as a gluten enteropathy. The condition is related in some way to the gluten found particularly in wheat and rye. There is a toxic portion (gliadin) which causes a hypersensitivity reaction and/or a local inflammatory reaction and pathological changes in the structure of the absorbing cells of the small intestine, leading to malabsorption. The symptoms are typical of the malabsorption syndrome. Manifestations include large foul-smelling, bulky, frothy and pale colored stools containing high fat content. There are usually recurrent attacks of diarrhea, with accompanying stomach cramps, alternating with constipation. There is often some edema and abdominal distention.

In many cases, elimination of gluten from the diet produces a dramatic improvement in symptoms and the restoration of normal function of the small intestine. This calls for avoiding all grains except corn and rice. However, amylase enzymes from plant sources of *Aspergillus niger* are effective *in vitro* in the treatment of celiac disease. By using this enzyme to cleave the toxic carbohydrate portion of the culprit gliadin fraction, the grains with gluten could be rendered harmless in susceptible individuals.

Those are just two examples of digestive enzyme insufficiency in otherwise normal people. But the case for supplementation is to be made, not from disease, but from the nutritional model. It is to do what is **normal, natural and necessary**. That is why you should put enzymes to work for you.

Animal derived digestive enzymes are often used as supplements. Pepsin is prepared from the stomach of pigs and another supplement is extracted from the pancreas of slaughter house animals. *Pepsin* supplements are sometimes used for patients with poor protein digestion and it works only in the highly acid medium of the stomach. It does nothing for fats and carbohydrates. *Pancreatic extracts* work on these in the alkaline intestines. In order to make them suitable for oral use they are made into so called enteric coated tablets. This protects them from the acid in the stomach en route. When they reach the intestine, the alkaline juice dissolves the coating and releases the enzymes. Again, they are used where the pancreas fails to make these enzymes.

A much better alternative to these animal derivatives is to use **plant enzymes derived from live cultures**. These can be obtained commercially today and they have much better bioactive profiles. They are called 'plant' enzymes but they function in the same manner as those enzymes indigenous to the human body. The source may be different but we are dealing with a totally organic, biological (live) cellular factory (not a synthetic laboratory) and the product is the same. More importantly, the bioactivity is no different. They work effectively in the food enzyme stomach where normal pre-digestion should take place. As we mentioned earlier, they also work at the various pH levels throughout the gastro-intestinal tract and also optimally at body temperature. They seem ideally designed for that very purpose.

Supplementation with these plant enzymes is the way to go to optimize digestion and to obtain the maximum benefit from the essential foods you eat. It provides, in principle, a guaranteed daily supply of these normal, natural and necessary ingredients of foods in a most convenient form.

ii) Systemic Enzymes for your body

Digestive enzymes are fairly easy to understand and appreciate. So that kind of supplementation has not seen much opposition from either the lay public or from the professional community, by and large. However, going beyond that is a much different matter. Enzyme function in metabolism and general physiology is perceived as something the human body does internally and independently - without any external help, thank you very much.

However, one of the more exciting recent developments in the field of complementary medicine has been the availability of orally ingestible systemic enzymes as a nutritional means to affect a wide variety of common conditions. It is even tempting to think medically again and to focus on therapeutic applications but that is for the specialists to deal with. For general purposes, you need only to appreciate the intrinsic value of this dietary consideration.

The increasing prevalence and wide range of documented research has demonstrated that systemic enzymes benefit specific conditions in the body. Much of this research has gone unrecognized by the mainstream health professionals because it is not intuitively plausible. Enzymes are usually thought of as very large, complex protein molecules that likely get degraded in the gut and therefore have little bioactive significance beyond the intestinal lumen or wall.

But not so. The direct opposite turns out to be the case. Many enzymes are indeed stable enough to resist acid and alkali destruction and they are still not too large to be absorbed through the "leaky bowel phenomenon", even in normal individuals. Yes, macromolecules can and do pass intact from the human gut into the blood stream under ordinary conditions.

In a nutshell, **pure plant enzymes, with typical molecular weights in the 35,000 range, are fully absorbed following oral administration.**

Other animal and human studies have shown that numerous specific whole proteins, including different plant and animal enzymes, are absorbed intact into the blood stream (5). These include surprisingly, human albumin and lactalbumin, bovine albumin, oralbumin, lactoglobulin, ferritin (imagine, with a molecular weight of 500,000), chymotripsinogen, elastase, and even other larger molecules such as botulism toxin (are you ready for this? -a molecular weight of 1,000,000!). Even inert particles, such as carbon particles from Indian Ink, and whole viruses too, can cross the healthy intestinal wall.

Even more dramatic is the finding that both the enzymes produced in the body, as well as supplementary enzymes and food enzymes, are not only absorbed intact from the gut, but they are also transported through the bloodstream, taken up intact by the pancreatic secretory cells and then re-secreted into the intestinal lumen by the pancreas and mixed with newly synthesized pancreatic juices (6). This circulation of proteolytic enzymes could be compared to similar recycling of bile salts by the liver.

So what exactly are these systemic enzymes? These are generally the same proteases, amylase and lipase found naturally in the body. Of course, the proteolytic enzymes like trypsin and chymotrypsin are of special interest because so much of the body biochemistry is orchestrated through protein molecules. If amino acids are letters of a cellular alphabet, then the proteins form words, sentences and complete paragraphs in cellular communication. If they were bricks, then the proteins would form walls to build amazing structures. Proteolytic enzymes in these metaphors, cleave the words and sentences to change the meaning and likewise dissolve the mortar between the bricks to tear down walls.

Systemic enzymes are obviously different from digestive enzymes. The latter work in the gut to break down large molecules into smaller molecules for absorption and later use in cellular synthesis. Systemic enzymes exert their beneficial effects at a local cellular level where they replenish, in advancing years, the declining reservoir of naturally occurring enzymes in cells. They break down proteins. They even do this in the circulation and in interstitial spaces in tissues and between cells.

There is apparent effectiveness of systemic enzyme therapy in the nutritional management of some clinical conditions. But again, we must not be distracted or diverted by such medical therapeutics. This is not primarily the subject of treatment but rather of **prevention.** The goal of nutrition must always be, first and foremost, to empower the body to protect itself. The body is engineered for preserving health and even promoting healing, if given adequate amounts of the right building blocks and all the right tools to do the job.

The building blocks are the amino acids found in food proteins; the free fatty acids available from the energy dense fats we eat; and the simple sugars for more immediate forms of energy, tied together in the form of carbohydrates. That's the basic stuff of which we are made. At the same time, we need all the essential foods - including enzymes, plus vitamins and minerals - to provide the necessary tools to complete the body's formidable armamentarium. Your job is to fill up that tool box and then stand back and watch your own body go to work. There is no one better for that job!

But how do you get the building materials to the construction sites and the tools into the box? That's the challenge of cellular nutrition. Enzymes hold the key, so it **really is a question of Enzyme Nutrition.**

That's next. It's another integral part of the foundation for applying **The Enzyme Diet™ Solution.**

ENZYME NUTRITION
A New Approach

You're Not What You Eat!

You're **not** what you eat! That's probably not what you'll think at first. The famous nutritionist Adelle Davis wrote a book years ago with the title: *You Are What You Eat.* She was close, inasmuch as she put the spotlight on the importance of nutrition. That was at a time when the agriculture food industry had given way to the industrial food era. Needless to say, if you change the quality and quantity of your food intake, you will become a reflection of that very shift.

But life has never been that simple. You're either much more or probably much less than what you put in your mouth. Let's consider your body as a construction site. You are building and re-building all the time. What you build there will always depend on your materials, the delivery system and the quality of workers and their tools. After all, what you eat is very important and sets a limit to both the length and quality of your life and health. However, the real variable is not what you eat, but rather **it's what your cells eat**! That's where the action really is.

The miracle of life - and in some ways, its secret - is the metabolic activity taking place all the time **inside** the living cell. We pointed out earlier that healthy cells make up healthy organs and tissues, and healthy organs make up healthy bodies. That cellular metabolic activity involves the consumption and turnover of indispensable nutrients obtained from the normal diet. Those same nutrients and the energy they provide must be present in the food you eat. That is where it all begins. But in real terms, that is only the beginning.

To use a different metaphor, think of your body as a donut. The hole in the donut represents your digestive tract. It really is that simple. What would go in the donut hole would not be in the donut itself, and similarly, what goes in the mouth to fill the stomach is not really inside the body per se. At least, not yet. It remains in an external space, at least as far as **the cells** are concerned. And that's what matters.

This is basic biology. It is fundamental **Food Science 101**. But it is often overlooked. Let's look at it again.

When you eat, you ingest food that enters a long hollow tube that traverses some thirty to forty feet -- end to end. This tube is a highly sophisticated corridor of life. It has many specialized systems and departments for a number of critical physiological activities. To name some of the most important ones, consider the following:

> • *Transportation of its contents by an involuntary process known as peristalsis.* When that fails, life is threatened. The clinical condition where nothing moves along is called an ileus. It has varied causes and is a constant challenge in the hospital, especially after surgery.
> • *Nerve centers for mostly involuntary (reflex) control.* This could be protective as in some forms of reflex vomiting or diarrhea. The wandering vagus nerve connects directly to the brain.
> • *Active hormone secretions and receptor sites for integration of many different body functions.* This is a primary gateway to the body and therefore, coordination of body needs and functions is crucial.
> • *Portals of entry for a variety of digestive juices and fluids.* Gastric secretions, pancreatic juices and bile fluids are all orchestrated for maximum efficiency.
> • *A complex immunological defense along its borders.* This protects the integrity of the intestinal wall and exerts some controlling influence as watchmen at the gate.

So it's sophisticated. But it is still a sophisticated hole, open at both ends and separated from the rest of your body by a wall. Entrance to the hole (the mouth) is what you control, but entrance to the donut (the body itself) is where the true discrimination takes place. There, nature takes over and you have little say in the matter.

In reality, the food that enters your mouth does not enter your body per se until different parts of it cross the intestinal wall and enter into the circulation. The blood then conducts the derived nutrients to all parts of your body, there to be utilized by individual cells. Those are the trillions of little building sites where the old you is constantly being protected and the new you is always under construction.

You Are Only What Your Cells Eat

When most people think of nutrition, they think only of the food they eat or the supplements they take. That is superficial and an inadequate oversimplification. The true definition of nutrition, however, is **to nourish the cells of the body in order to optimize their metabolism for optimum health and provide energy to live.** This is **Cellular Nutrition.**

Cellular nutrition does not happen automatically or inevitably, but instead requires several complex steps. These processes can be simplified into the **"Seven Steps of Nutrition"**:

1. Ingestion: *The addition of food or supplements into the intestinal lumen,* usually through the mouth. This is the only voluntary step. If you fail to eat what you need, there is not much that your body can do. Adequate intake is indispensable.

2. Digestion: *The process of converting complex food into simple molecules* that can be easily absorbed through the intestine into the blood. This is a continuous process, beginning in the mouth but mainly taking place in the stomach and the early part of the small intestine. If you fail to digest, malabsorption takes place and symptoms follow.

3. Absorption: *The transfer of substances from the intestinal lumen* across the wall and into the circulation for transport throughout the body. Malabsorption of any class of nutrients can have dire clinical consequences.

4. Circulation: *The transport of nutrients from the intestine to the cells of the body,* mainly via the bloodstream. Most of these are stable but some require special carriers, usually by serum proteins.

5. Assimilation: *The transfer of nutrients from the circulation into the cells of the body.* The nutrients must cross over the sophisticated cell-wall barrier (membrane) and enter the cell itself, where the real action takes place inside. Remember that critical axiom: cells self-serve. They feed like little piglets from the circulating trough.

6. Metabolism: *The sum total of all the biochemical processes that occur in each cell* of the body, and which are required for life. There are thousands - perhaps millions - of different chemical and physiological changes taking place every second inside these trillions of microscopic cells. Therein is the mystery of life itself. No human mind can fathom that awesome complexity. It works only when all the parts and workers are present.

7. Detoxification: *The removal of metabolic waste products and toxins from the body.* Those follow a reverse pathway where the waste products of metabolism leave the cells to enter the circulation again. This time they go via the liver, usually for conversion to more harmless products, which are then excreted via the filtration system of the kidney. Undigested waste is eliminated at the end of the intestinal lumen.

These seven basic steps were designed by nature, not science, and are all essential for complete cellular nutrition to occur. When any of these steps does not function correctly, nutrients will not be effectively delivered to the cells of the body. As a result, healthy metabolism will not be maintained and disease will usually occur. If left untreated (or better still, unmanaged) the ultimate consequence is death. We therefore eat to live!

Unfortunately, most people take the majority of these steps for granted even when they eat. We have a meal and immediately forget it. The rest becomes history. Yet one cannot overstate that it is not just what we eat, but what we at least digest, absorb, assimilate and metabolize that determines our health. Many people, even those concerned with "eating right," don't realize the importance of ensuring that the nutrients in foods are available to the individual cells. Do you?

Even supplement formulators have forgotten this important principle. They concoct their **nutritional supplements** without much thought of how to literally supplement, or add to, the nutrition the body's cells receive. To truly nourish the body, the nutrients must not merely be ingested, but must be digested and assimilated - broken down and delivered to the individual cells of the body. It is on the cellular level that the body is nourished, regenerated and supplied with fuel for proper functioning.

Just imagine the vast quantities of nutrients being flushed daily through the bodies of millions of people who neglect these important considerations - even if with the best of intentions. Many people eat too much, but the **quantity** of food/calories is not the issue. Those people who supplement their diet with valuable nutrients to improve health and wellness, but again, without effective delivery to the cells, derive only limited benefit. No matter what good intentions one has, nutritious and expensive waste is still waste. You need to think of your delivery system.

However, it has become very popular throughout the world to add supplements to the diet to improve overall nutrition. This has come about as most of the specialists in health science and now medicine, have become increasingly aware of the limitations of modern diets and the very important links between nutrition and health and disease. This is no longer debatable. The evidence is clearly overwhelming. So the practice of food supplementation in all its forms and varieties is here to stay.

But even taking nutritional supplements is just one limited thing. Being sure that the nutrients desired are actually delivered to and used by each and every cell of your body is quite another. That will be only a product of design, not default.

The situation may be even worse than it appears. Many nutritional supplements actually "rob" other nutrient factors from the body while trying to perform their work. Why? Every time you put a nutrient into your body, it requires other nutritional co-factors (especially vitamins and minerals) in order to work effectively. That demand can therefore deplete those same essential co-factors which may be required for more vital physiologic functions at any given time.

We have been conditioned by the media and the current 'health and wellness' mentality to make sure that we take our vitamins and minerals every day. That's fine. We are rightly encouraged to eat lots of fruits and vegetables and take good supplements too. No argument there. But we hardly ever hear the recommendation to take any enzymes or replenish our enzyme reserves. However, we lose more of these daily than we do of the vitamins and minerals. Enzymes are far more easily burned up and used up than vitamins and minerals. And remember, the enzymes are the true stars after all.

When you stop to think about it, the need to supplement with enzymes may be greater than the need for supplementary vitamins and minerals. Yet, many thousands of books, articles and research papers, sponsored and published, or approved by the drug companies that process and manufacture vitamins, continue to suggest, (if not to claim) that isolated, refined vitamins are capable of normalizing body physiology and even having therapeutic effects on some diseases.

But every scientific manual which goes to the core of vitamin biochemistry, spells out clearly what we already emphasized in the last chapter - that **vitamins are merely enzyme activators and catalysts**. They have but this one central function and role. When inside our bodies, each vitamin works only when in conjunction with specific enzymes. By previous analogy, enzymes are the true stars, while vitamins and minerals are the support players.

Our body's requirements for living are enormous and isolated enzymes are slow, sluggish workers. By themselves, they are incapable of keeping up with the body's needs for fuel and energy, and the creation and restoration of structural materials. They cannot bring about all the changes and supply all the body's needs, as fast as our daily activities and living require them. They need their vitamin and mineral activators/accelerators. Vitamins and minerals are co-enzymes that increase the rate and efficiency of enzyme productivity.

In effect then, if all the necessary co-factors are not provided with any supplement itself, that supplement "leaches" the co-factors from your body, depriving you of the nutrient factors you already had in storage! These nutrients could have been used to help repair damaged cells, make new cells, prevent disease and provide you with the energy you need to feel and look younger. Therefore, you could in principle, be doing more harm than good by taking a supplement without an effective system for nutrient delivery. It's that simple and that important too!

Your important focus of nutrition must therefore be always on *cellular nutrition*. There is no other way to truly satisfy your body's needs.

That presents a challenge ...

స్

A Nutrient Delivery System

Years ago, the scientists at Infinity2 Inc. in Arizona foresaw that the future of human nutrition would be in this cellular delivery. That is, they recognized how important it was that the nutrients in your food and the supplements you swallow be fully used by your body and not just simply passed through. They must be guaranteed to get out of the hole and into the donut, as it were. Nobody had been successful in figuring out how to get that done until the Infinity2 specialists made their breakthrough.

The Formulation Team at Infinity2, led by their Senior Director, the late biochemist **Dr. Stan Bynum,** spent years researching the way Nature designed nutrients to be delivered. Their studies finally unlocked the secret of how to recreate Nature's own delivery process. Using the most leading-edge, all-natural, biomedical science, Infinity2 created an original and effective nutrient delivery system.

This innovative system is called **CAeDS®** - an abbreviated acronym for the original Chelate Activated Enzyme Delivery System. This system ensures that nutrients are absorbed and delivered to your cells, which after all is their ultimate destination. It is all natural, exclusive to Infinity2 and in everything they make.

That includes **The Enzyme Diet™**. In its weight loss application, it is critical that your cells get the adequate nutrients they need. They must satisfy their metabolic requirements and maintain your basic metabolic rate even while you lose weight. Only satisfied cells can allow you to retain good health and energetic feelings, both during the active weight loss program and after you attain your desired goal and work to keep it there.

CAeDS® is a highly refined and sophisticated system that provides the necessary nutritional co-factors and patented amino-acid-chelated minerals for full activation and assimilation of all the nutrients you consume as food or supplements. And it is designed to do all this, without "robbing" from your body's limited supply!

CAeDS® is still the same exclusive process developed by Dr. Bynum and his colleagues, using the basic principles first given to them directly by **Dr. Edward Howell**, the discoverer of Enzyme Nutrition whom we referred to repeatedly in the last chapter. Dr. Howell was also the founder of his own company, which became a leader in research and commercial manufacture of plant enzymes for widespread use. You will recall his practical Enzyme Nutrition principle from the last chapter: **a full complement of digestive enzymes must be ingested along with food for the complete nutritional value of the food to be delivered to the cells of the body**. Dr. Howell's research provided the background to precisely coordinate the nutrients in any supplement formula, with the exact combination of enzymes required to deliver those nutrients to the cells of the body. The process, identified and utilized by Infinity2 scientists in formulating their breakthrough design, is known as **Enzyme Delivery**. This innovative Enzyme Delivery has made it possible to make natural supplements with the essential characteristics of whole, fresh food.

In order for each of the seven steps of nutrition to function properly, specific enzymes are required. For example, adequate **Digestive Enzymes** must be present in order for food to be converted or broken down into the useful nutrients that can be absorbed. But are they? And are they sufficient? What are some of the determining factors?

All fruits, vegetables and herbs have a specific chemical composition. Sometimes this can occlude or hold on to the desired nutrients making either digestion or absorption more difficult than it might otherwise be. This chemical composition and the ability of the body to digest or break it down can affect the availability of the nutrients contained within the food. For example:

· *Proteins* can bind certain vitamins and minerals (take calcium, for example) and decrease their absorption. There's an illustration of how standard food labels and textbook nutritional data could be misleading.
· *Complex carbohydrates* can bind minerals, proteins and other nutrients, thereby also limiting bioavailability. This negates the minimal value of the 'tea and toast' diet of so many seniors.

· *Fats* and oils coat some nutrients, again decreasing their level of absorption. That's the downside, for fat digestion and absorption normally allows the fat-soluble vitamins A, D, E and K to be absorbed effectively.

In summary, it has been shown that **alteration of the macromolecular structure of foods and herbs can improve the release of vitamins, minerals and phytonutrients.**

This alteration of the macromolecular structure of foods and herbs occurs through the action of a variety of digestive enzymes. This process occurs naturally in the body under normal circumstances. However, stress, environmental toxins, cooking and processing of foods, disease conditions, aging etc. effectively deplete digestive enzyme action and can prevent this process from occurring properly. We saw at the end of the last chapter how, in principle, you can put digestive enzymes to work for you by careful supplementation with plant enzymes. This would be *normal, natural and necessary*. Clearly, exogenous digestive enzymes derived from natural fermentation cultures could be ingested along with food to optimize this process.

So much for digestive enzymes - that's the first component of CAeDS®. There's more.

Absorption and assimilation of nutrients both require one or more of several **Membrane-transport Enzymes**. These enzymes are complex, highly specific and critical (as all enzymes are). They facilitate passage through the intestinal cell walls and across each individual cell membrane throughout the body. Without these enzymes, nutrients cannot be delivered to the cells of the body. In other words, the nutritional value of food and supplements would be lost without these sophisticated enzymes.

Such specialized enzymes are even more specific as to which nutrients they metabolize and transport. In addition, they require co-factors to function optimally. The body's natural processes call for coordinated enzymes and minerals to be present in order for nutrients to be delivered to the individual cells. As a net result, a number of specific **Minerals and Co-factors** must be present in order for maximum enzyme activity to occur. Without these necessary co-factors, essential enzyme activity robs the body's nutrient stores. That consideration led to a further development.

The next breakthrough therefore came when the Infinity2 Formulation Team led by Dr. Stan Bynum, compared the enzyme work of Dr. Edward Howell with that of the internationally acclaimed, mineral nutrition scientist, **Dr. Harvey Ashmead**. He became the third star to complete the professional trio that gave birth to CAeDS®. Dr. Ashmead authored a classic book in his field: *Intestinal Absorption of Metal Ions and Chelates* (Charles C. Thomas: Springfield, 1985). His son, H. DeWayne Ashmead, also a Ph.D. nutritionist and expert in the same field, later edited *The Roles of Amino Acid Chelates in Animal Nutrition* (Noyes Publications, 1993) to further underscore the importance of this research area. With their extensive knowledge and research experience, together they ranked among the world's leading authorities on chelated minerals. Their research into methods of bonding amino acids to minerals resulted in the multi-patented chelated mineral process and produced the most efficiently assimilated form of mineral supplementation available anywhere.

Dr. Harvey Ashmead (father) founded Albion International, Inc. in 1956 and was its President for many years. Albion became one of the world's leaders in research and manufacturing of bioactive chelated minerals. Today, Dr. H. DeWayne Ashmead (son) serves as its current president. No other company has gone to the extent that Albion has to ensure that minerals are absorbed and available for use in the body. They were true pioneers in the field of mineral nutrition.

When minerals such as zinc, magnesium, iron and others become surrounded by *and bonded to* amino acids, *in a stable form*, this is true chelation. It provides a natural means for the body to effectively transport minerals across the intestinal wall. These chelates also remain stable in the circulation and become active even in the processes of cellular metabolism.

Dr. Harvey Ashmead, in consulting with Infinity2's formulators, expressed how excited he was with the use of enzymes in nutritional formulas. He also repeatedly emphasized that enzymes do require specific minerals as co-factors to reach their full activity. Infinity2's formulation team soon realized that the highest level of nutrient delivery could only be achieved by utilizing Dr. Ashmead's chelated minerals as co-factors in the enzyme delivery system. This became the second major component of the CAeDS® innovative formulation. Now you can clearly appreciate the acronym for what it really means:

CAeDS® - *The Chelate Activated Enzyme Delivery System*

There you have it. To put it another way: chelates activate enzymes and that makes the delivery system complete. Building upon the basis of the *enzyme* research done by pioneer researcher Dr. Edward Howell and then *activating* them with the *chelated* mineral research done by the innovative researcher Dr. Harvey Ashmead, another outstanding scientist, Dr. Stan Bynum, was able to lead his formulation team to create the CAeDS® *delivery system* for Infinity2. No other company in the world uses this proprietary method of formulation. It is a true classic.

Always a visionary, Dr. Bynum modified the original enzyme delivery system by incorporating additional enzymes when most appropriate. In addition, he utilized only the readily absorbed and chemically proven chelated minerals from Albion, to assure maximum enzyme activation. These patented chelated minerals from the Albion laboratories are without competition in the industry. Thus, CAeDS® has become a premium system of nutrient delivery.

The CAeDS® trademark name refers to a combination of ingredients, which ensure that each of the products commercialized by Infinity2 are bioavailable, absorbed and transported to the cells with maximum efficiency. CAeDS® brings to Infinity2 formulations the highest level of nutrient delivery yet achieved in nutritional supplementation. This is the delivery system utilized in **The Enzyme Diet™** to maximize the benefit of all the nutrients provided to the cells. Even during a weight loss exercise, the focus must still be on cellular nutrition. In fact, particularly so, since satisfied cells will maintain metabolism to avert the undesirable reactive consequences we saw earlier. This leads to personal satisfaction, high energy and vitality, and therefore good compliance.

CAeDS® provides the necessary minerals and co-factors for optimum enzyme activity without robbing vital nutrients from the body. CAeDS® utilizes the principle of close coordination of enzyme activity with specific levels of chelated minerals, and with the nutrient content of the formula. The enzymes in CAeDS® are precisely coordinated with the nutrients in **The Enzyme Diet™** to achieve optimum delivery of the nutrients.

By way of summary then, the function of CAeDS® is based on the following five principles:

1. **The true definition of nutrition is to nourish the cells of the body - cellular nutrition**. In order for cellular nutrition to occur, several complex steps must occur. These are in order: ingestion, digestion, absorption, circulation, assimilation, metabolism and detoxification.

2. **Specific enzymes are required for these steps to occur optimally**. These include digestive enzymes and essential co-factors. Enzymes consist of complex proteins that require one or more minerals as co-factors to express their activity.

3. **Amino Acid Chelates are the most bioavailable and best-utilized form of minerals**. The term "amino acid chelates" refers to the product resulting from the reaction of one or more amino acids with a metal ion, which results in a chemically bonded compound with a total molecular weight of 1,000 Daltons or less. When done properly, chelation of the mineral with appropriate amino acids enhances mineral bioavailability.

4. **CAeDS® is matched to nature**. CAeDS® combines the patented Albion Chelated Minerals with specific enzymes to create a delivery system capable of ensuring that the nutrients found in foods and supplements are effectively delivered to the cells of the body. CAeDS® ensures that the necessary co-factors are matched to the exact balance found in nature.

5. **Supplements should be non-toxic**. The ingredients in a supplement should not create products which cannot be utilized by the body. Amino acid chelates are sufficiently stable, and when properly formulated, are absorbed unchanged into biological systems where the chelate is transported to the site of utilization. At that site, the chelate bond can be enzymatically broken and the mineral ion and amino acids may be used separately by the system. The enzymes in CAeDS® are also broken down in this same way to minerals and amino acids which can then participate in metabolism as nutrients also.

These are the basic concepts behind the formulation of CAeDS®. This guaranteed delivery system is based on a combination of the research of the enzymologist Dr. Howell, and the research and patents of Albion Laboratories, including **US Patent #5,882,685** relating to **the use of amino acid chelated minerals in increasing enzyme activity,** and **US Patent #4,863,898** related to the **tissue-specific delivery of nutrients.**

These two patents, by themselves, combine to make this proprietary technology most credible to the individual consumer and should reassure both professional and lay public alike. Patents are not just ideas, they are demonstrated *reductions to practice* with all the necessary supporting evidence and documentation to justify attendant claims. They are available for scrutiny in the public domain. Just look at the Titles and the Abstracts and put two and two together.

US Patent #5,882,685:   Food energy utilization from carbohydrates in animals

Abstract

A method for facilitating digestion of carbohydrates into simple sugars in warm-blooded animals by maintaining and enhancing the natural disaccharidase enzymatic activity in the mucosal cells of the small intestines. Iron is an essential mineral and other minerals selected from the group consisting of copper, zinc, manganese and cobalt are provided in the form of amino acid chelates having a ligand to mineral molar ratio of at least 1:1, a molecular weight of no more than 1500 daltons and a stability constant of between about 10.sup.6 and 10.sup.16 and administered orally. Additionally, magnesium and chromium, as amino acid chelates, may be added to improve disaccharidase activity as may potassium in inorganic salt form or as a 1:1 ligand to potassium amino acid complex. The minerals are taken into the mucosal cells lining the small intestine where they are utilized to facilitate the production and activity of disaccharidase enzymes such as maltase, sucrase and lactase. These enzymes promote the hydrolysis of disaccharides resulting from degradation of more complex carbohydrates or of sucrose and lactose into simple sugars or monosaccharides for absorption from the intestinal tract.

US Patent #4,863,898:   Amino acid chelated compositions for delivery to specific biological tissue sites

Abstract

Amino acid chelates having a ligand to divalent metal mole ratio of at least 2:1 and having a molecular weight of not more than 1500 and preferably not more than 1000 and also having a stability constant of between about 10.sup.6 and 10.sup.16 are formulated for delivery to one or more specific tissue sites within a mammal. The ligand utilized in formulating the amino acid chelate is a naturally occuring amino acid or a dipeptide, tripeptide or quadrapeptide thereof. The selection of an appropriate ligand with which to form the chelate provides a product that, when entering the bloodstream of the mammal, either by mean of oral ingestion or injection, has a propensity to migrate to one or more targeted tissue sites within the mammal.

The first patent demonstrates the first claim of using amino acid chelates to activate enzymes. Similarly the second one demonstrates the efficacy of specific tissue delivery of nutrients. Put together, that's the basic principle of CAeDS® in a nutshell.

Note: If you're interested in the more detailed science behind CAeDS®, a more thorough discussion is given in the Appendix 'A'.

CAeDS® cellular delivery is one comprehensive concept that sets **The Enzyme Diet™** apart. This unique Meal Replacement Superfood formulation has been designed to deliver cellular nutrition to effectively impact metabolism. No other meal replacement available can make that substantial claim. Throughout the formulation process, Infinity2 looked at what actually gets into and is used by the body.

As in all other aspects of micro-nutrition, quality is everything. At the cellular level, only rigorous standards of excellence based on nature and good science will do. Obviously, paid advertising, packaging and pricing strategies make no appeal to cells. Cells cannot be distracted by 'smoke and mirrors,' or deceived by slight of hand, but they can be influenced by science at its best.

This exclusive system has been proven to deliver nutrients to the cells of the body in total harmony with the body's own mechanisms. With CAeDS® included, **The Enzyme Diet™** is able to supply the highest level of nutrient delivery yet achieved by supplementation. The Infinity2 company has gone to these lengths to ensure that supplementation provides you with every nutritional component your body needs, and more importantly, **at the cellular level**. This is a crucial consideration for effective weight loss if it is to stay lost.

❧

CAeDS® SUMMARY

CAeDS® - The Chelate-Activated Enzyme Delivery System - is Infinity2's proprietary method of formulating products to increase the bioavailability of nutrients and phytochemicals from whole foods and herbs. It is an exclusive process developed by the Infinity2, Inc. Product Formulation Team using the principles first elucidated by Dr. Edward Howell, the discoverer of Enzyme Nutrition.

The body's natural processes call for coordinated enzymes and minerals to be present in order for nutrients to be delivered to the cells of the body. With CAeDS®, the Infinity2 scientists have been able to provide the same balance that exists in nature. Certain specific minerals and co-factors must be present in order for enzyme activity to occur. The patented Albion amino acid chelated minerals are used to fully activate the enzymes, thereby producing a unique delivery system. Without these necessary co-factors, enzyme activity could rob the body's nutrient stores.

And finally, what's the bottomline? **The CAeDS® System impacts each of the seven steps to cellular nutrition.**

CAeDS®:

· **Protects nutrients from toxins in the intestinal lumen.**

· **Provides enzymes required for digestion.**

· **Provides enzymes and anti-oxidants to protect nutrients during transport to cells.**

· **Provides enzymes and nutrient co-factors required for transport across cell membranes.**

· **Provides nutrient co-factors required for optimum function of the membrane-transport enzymes of the cells.**

· **Provides amino acids, vitamins and minerals for metabolic processes after the role of delivery is complete.**

· **Ingredients are non-toxic and add no burden to the detoxification processes of the body.**

When all is said and done, you can now benefit from this effective nutrient delivery system. It is an active ingredient of **The Enzyme Diet™** meal replacement formulation and assures the optimum delivery of all the fine nutrients it provides.

And why is this so important?

During usual weight loss, cells are threatened by starvation. Metabolism slows. Dieters experience the typical symptoms like hunger, weakness, headache and lethargy. Then there is the problem of rebound. Sooner, more often than later, the weight creeps back, then frustration and poor compliance follow. It all ends in failure and disappointment.

So what's the answer?

You guessed it! **The Enzyme Diet™** is a low-fat, nutrient-dense Superfood, ideally suited as a meal replacement in a comprehensive program designed for effective weight loss. It supplies the nutrients needed to support the body's metabolism. The power of its enzymes and co-factors ensures that the nutrients needed for optimum metabolism are delivered to the cells of the body.

The Enzyme Diet™ could be just the solution you need. You can now shed unwanted pounds as fat, retain and build your lean muscle and improve your general state of health, all at the same time. It is discussed in detail in the next chapter.

❧ *Chapter 6* ❧

THE ENZYME DIET
A New Alternative

We began this book with a look at the burdensome problem of overweight and obesity in America. You recall that The Surgeon General has recently focused on this silent epidemic as a national crisis and issued a call to action for all levels of society to make some necessary changes to reduce not just the weight of Americans, but the dangerous and costly health consequences. In Chapter 2 we made a selective review of some of the more popular diets and weight loss programs that together have proven to be an elusive remedy. Some 90-95% of participants have experienced the frustration of watching any quick substantial reduction in their weight lead to a rebound within a year or two. But Americans continue to search, to spend and to hope for some practical solution to their weight dilemma.

We looked a little deeper in Chapter 3 to find out what could be the crux of the problem. We know that there probably is some genetic predisposition which might influence a set point or range for each individual to be stable, even with disadvantages to health in many cases. We also know that we have created in our affluent society, a toxic environment that works against the best intentions to keep one's weight under control. We have an over abundance of high calorie foods, especially the ever present, fast and convenient foods that the industry keeps pushing on the gullible public. At the same time, technology has changed our culture into a sedentary lifestyle of ease and entertainment, where even our children are not getting exposed to adequate physical activity. Nevertheless, the *energy (calorie) balance equation* still holds true. If you consume more energy as calories in food and expend less in exercise, the net difference is what you will always store as fat. So the ideal weight loss program still calls for you to reduce calorie consumption and increase your exercise to experience effective weight loss that stays lost.

But is there a real solution? Can you reduce your calorie intake to favor the burning of excess fat and yet satisfy your cells' needs and maintain essential metabolism? Is it possible to diet in this way and yet feel satisfied, energetic and even enjoy better health at the same time? Can you lose weight and have it remain lost?

The answer to all these questions is a resounding YES! So we began the second section of this book with a look at the all important but often neglected basis of all our metabolic activity. A new awareness probably dawned on you as you looked at the secret of all physical life. The emphasis on enzymes as the indispensable work force of your body led you to realize that they are more than just catalysts to be taken for granted. These highly sophisticated protein molecules are most precious in nature and constitute what Dr. Leo Roy called *the life of life*.

Thanks to the life's work of Dr.Edward Howell, we now have a new biological appreciation for enzyme nutrition. Hopefully, you now understand the Food Enzyme Concept and appreciate the importance of ensuring adequate dietary intake of enzymes in food and supplements to effectively spare your body's enzyme potential. In this way you leave your A-team players, all those fine metabolic enzymes that your cells synthesize, to do what they do best. In fact, they will then do what only they can do. That is, they maintain proper levels of metabolism even as you attempt to lose weight and keep it off.

You can **put enzymes to work for you** to get the healthy and permanent results that you desire. You can include supplementary digestive enzymes to ensure the optimum digestion of all your precious dietary intake and maximum absorption of those essential nutrients. You can supercharge your metabolism or better still, you can allow your cells to do what they really want to do.

But you also need **an adequate supply of all the essential nutrients** to build those metabolic enzymes and to give the cells the raw materials for growth and repair as well as for energy and defense. That's where the new approach to cellular nutrition becomes so very important. Not only do you need the components made up of amino acids, simple sugars and the essential free fatty acids, plus all the essential vitamins and minerals that you hear so much talk about, but you need an effective delivery system to get those nutrients inside your cells where they belong. The key is to exploit the synergy of supplementary amino acid chelates and enzymes to impact each step of cellular nutrition. That defines a delivery system - **an effective nutrient delivery system.** That's why CAeDS® makes such a big difference. This innovative chelate-activated enzyme delivery system takes supplementation to a whole new level. Now you can truly impact your cellular nutrition at all seven essential steps from ingestion and digestion, through absorption, assimilation and circulation, to the final metabolism and ultimate detoxification.

That recap should all make sense to you by now.

As you might expect, if you put all three **Key Elements** together, you'll have a winning solution. So here's the plan:

1. **Put those Enzymes - *the life of life* - to work for you;**

2. **Include all the Essential Nutrients your cells need;**

3. **Package them with an Effective Delivery System -**

all as a tasty meal replacement and Superfood - and voilà, you'll then have **The Enzyme Diet™.**

This brings us then to the new alternative that we have been referring to throughout the book so far. In this chapter, you will be introduced to **The Enzyme Diet™** itself as **the solution to the missing link in the weight loss industry**. In the third and final section of the book, we will go on to describe in detail your personal application of **The Enzyme Diet™**. That will include developing your own plan, designing your own menu (complete with recipes for major meals and snacks), and then of course, determining your own necessary exercise program. With this application you'll soon have reason to take pride in your healthy, reduced body and your expanded mind. You will discover and come to admire the new amazing wonderful You and to celebrate life!

☙

Fifteen Years in
Design and Development

The Enzyme Diet™ did not come about just like that. It is the product of years of fine research and innovative thinking. If Dr. Edward Howell can be regarded as the originator of the essential enzyme ideas that constitute this new approach, and if Dr. Harvey Ashmead made amino acid chelates effective cofactors to potentiate the enzymes, then Dr. Stan Bynum should be acknowledged as the leader of the formulation team at Infinity2 Inc. which spent years in development to bring this final product to market.

Obviously, **The Enzyme Diet**™ brings together a number of technological advances that together create a synergy to allow this single Meal Replacement Superfood product to fulfil a variety of nutritional challenges. In a nutshell, you can now use the amazing power of enzymes to finally obtain the leaner and healthier body you desire.

We saw back in Chapter 2 that the use of **Meal Replacements** as a method for weight loss is not only practical and convenient but it is demonstrably effective. Here are at least **Ten Good Reasons** why you should choose this method for yourself:

1. **You have no need for tedious caloric calculations and adequate meal designs.**
2. **You retain some degree of flexibility and control.**
3. **You have the added convenience to accommodate your hectic schedule and lifestyle.**
4. **You gain all the essential nutrients and more without the caloric burden.**
5. **You still eat a varied and sensible dinner to satisfy your need for bulk and sensual delights.**
6. **You contend easily with eating on the road and on the run.**
7. **You can scale your intake up or down in response to real need.**
8. **You can easily flavor your meal replacement for variety and personal taste.**
9. **You can start or stop your diet at any time.**
10. **You need little adjustment to a lifelong maintenance program.**

The Enzyme Diet™ was designed as a delicious, healthy, low fat meal replacement shake for safe and responsible weight loss that could last a life time. When combined with a healthy active lifestyle and balanced eating, it will provide your body with everything it needs to support your metabolism, to sustain or improve your health and to conveniently lose weight. The goal is finally to provide effective weight loss that stays lost.

How will The Enzyme Diet™ help you lose weight?

As we have seen, the problem with typical low-calorie diets is that the body senses a shortage of nutrients for making energy, so it compensates by slowing metabolism. Most dieters then stop losing weight, even if they are eating almost nothing. In addition, a slowed metabolism causes the overwhelming majority to actually gain it back, and it is not uncommon for many to gain back more weight than they actually lost. However, **The Enzyme Diet™** is different:

- **FIRST**, The Enzyme Diet™ uses the potential of enzymes to support your metabolism without drugs or stimulants. It's like a "metabolic makeover", setting the stage for your body to pull fat from storage and use it as fuel, instead of going into the starvation mode as happens with so many other popular diets.

- **SECOND**, The Enzyme Diet™ also addresses this challenge by avoiding empty calories, while providing your body with all the necessary nutrients to satisfy your cells' needs and to keep its metabolic systems running at optimal rates.

- **THIRD**, The Enzyme Diet™ includes the exclusive CAeDS® system which ensures that these nutrients are delivered to each cell in your body.

You can say then, that the take home message is simply: that **The Enzyme Diet™** has three clearly distinct advantages for you. **It is able to Boost, to Feed and to Deliver, all at the same time.**

Advantage #1:   ENZYMES TO BOOST

It has **Plant Enzymes and co-factors** to maintain your metabolism as you lose weight - ie. a powerful makeover **"boost"**,

Advantage #2:   ESSENTIAL NUTRIENTS TO FEED

It has **Complete (natural-source) Nutrients** to feed your cells so they remain healthy and you don't starve - ie. a satisfying **"meal"**, and

Advantage #3:   AN EFFECTIVE SYSTEM TO DELIVER

It has an **Effective Delivery System** to get them all there, with maximum efficiency - ie. an effective **"dunk."**

Here's another word picture of three components to remember:

1.   **ENZYMES**
+
2.   **ESSENTIAL NUTRIENTS**
+
3.   **EFFECTIVE DELIVERY SYSTEM**

=   **THE ENZYME DIET™**

As such, **The Enzyme Diet™** is one of a kind. It is a Triple-E solution.   It is safe, effective and very convenient. It is derived from nature, formulated with science and tailored for you. It offers hope for a solution to the weight loss challenge.

The Enzyme Diet™ Solution utilizes this fine meal replacement product in a comprehensive program that allows you, the dieter, to lose weight effectively and to remain healthy and energetic at the same time. Finally, here's a practical solution where weight loss stays lost because it addresses the real crux of the problem.

☙

☙   The Enzyme Diet™ Solution   ☙

Now, here's the basic design or outline of **The Enzyme Diet™ Solution** (your personal application will be discussed in the next chapter). **It's as easy as 1-2-3**:

1.

To Lose weight the healthy way:
You should replace two meals a day, each with a delicious Enzyme Diet™ shake. Then eat a sensible third meal, designed for completeness and balance.

2.

To maintain your lean muscle mass:
You should exercise daily for 30 minutes or more, drink plenty of water (8 glasses per day) and enjoy fresh fruits or raw vegetables as snacks.

3.

To maintain your weight loss:
You should then replace one meal a day with a delicious Enzyme Diet™ shake and eat sensibly the rest of the day. If you gain a few pounds, return to the weight loss plan (repeat actions 1 and 2) until you reach your desired weight.

If you want to lose weight and you are under 18, pregnant, nursing, following a diet recommended by a doctor, have health problems or want to lose more than 30 pounds, you should see a doctor before starting this or any other diet. Aim not to lose much more than two pounds a week after the first week. Rapid weight loss may cause health problems. Do not use as a sole source of nutrition. Eat at least 1,200 calories a day.

Superfood

The intent of Dr. Bynum and his colleagues was not just to develop a meal replacement for effective weight loss per se. That fulfils a real need in any case. But to do that very thing, one still must provide adequate nutrition for cells. The result is obvious therefore, that a carefully designed meal replacement will itself be a kind of *Superfood* and that is essentially what **The Enzyme Diet™** is. It is packed with good natural source, healthy ingredients that will deliver, if you like, *secondary* benefits to the dieter.

Let's look at some of these.

1. A Nutrient Smorgasbord. You realize that **The Enzyme Diet™** is more than just a diet. It is an excellent natural source of protein, vitamins A and C, zinc, selenium, copper, manganese, chromium and molybdenum. It is also a good source of fiber, iron and magnesium. Because these nutrients are all derived from natural ingredients, there are traces of many other nutrients that are found naturally in foods and they complement the nutrient package.

The Enzyme Diet™ includes all the known necessary nutrients to support the body's metabolic enzymes, and also provides the digestive enzymes necessary to ensure that these nutrients are absorbed and delivered to the cells with maximum efficiency. It is the only meal replacement shake that utilizes patented amino acid chelated minerals for enhanced absorption and assimilation.

2. Soy Protein. It has been shown that 25 grams of soy protein on a daily basis, as part of a diet low in saturated fat and cholesterol, may reduce the risk of heart disease. Each serving of **The Enzyme Diet™** supplies 13 grams of soy protein for this and all the other heralded benefits of soy protein. As a good source of protein, **The Enzyme Diet™** is also free of saturated fat and cholesterol, with only a mere 2 grams of total fat per serving. The Enzyme Diet™ actually meets the American Heart Association food criteria for saturated fat and cholesterol for healthy people over the age of two years.

Soy is an excellent source of high quality protein. It is one of the oldest foods known to man and has been a staple of Asian diets for centuries. In fact, soy is a complete protein, equal in quality to meat, milk and egg protein. It provides *all* the essential amino acids.

The soy protein in **The Enzyme Diet**™ is from a non-genetically modified source (non-GMO) and is the highest quality soy protein available anywhere. The proteins are processed with water wash (rather than the common alcohol wash) which maintains the integrity of the naturally occurring amino acids, vitamins, minerals and other bioactive components. It is manufactured under strict specifications in order to guarantee a consistent, high-quality protein.

3. Inulin as a good source of fiber. Fiber is an often neglected but essential ingredient of any complete diet. **The Enzyme Diet**™ contains 2.7 grams per serving of a unique fiber source called inulin. Researchers have found that inulin contains some relatively low molecular weight carbohydrates called fructooligosaccharides which promote healthy digestion and the growth of friendly bacteria. They may also improve the absorption of several nutrients.

Soluble fiber like inulin absorbs water. Oatmeal gets gooey because the soluble fiber holds water. The same goes for split peas and dried beans. This quality provides a benefit that may help to lower blood cholesterol and stabilize blood glucose. Soluble fiber forms a gel, and as the gel moves through the intestines, it absorbs bile and delays the absorption of glucose. Bile is a digestive juice that is made by the liver. It normally is reused over and over again, but when it gets trapped in the soluble fiber gel, it is eliminated with the rest of the digestive waste products. In other words, it's flushed down the toilet. The liver will need to make more bile to replace what was lost. The liver uses cholesterol out of the bloodstream to make bile. Using cholesterol out of your bloodstream to make new bile means that your body cholesterol level is lowered. Soluble fiber also plays a role in keeping your intestine and colon healthy.

The Enzyme Diet™ is a good source of fiber. Each serving provides about 4 grams of fiber, primarily from soluble fibers. Snacking on fresh fruits and raw vegetables while on the plan, plus a sensible dinner choice, will allow you to meet your daily fiber requirement for sure. That's healthy.

4. Plant Enzymes.   It is important to remember that **The Enzyme Diet**™ contains a mixture of plant enzymes which were selected for their distinct advantages. It is well known that many of the enzymes derived from plants possess unusually high stability and activity under *a broad range of pH conditions*. These properties distinguish them from animal enzymes such as pepsin, pancreatin, trypsin and others, which require pH conditions often lacking in people with impaired health. For example, pepsin is active only below a pH of about 4.5 while pancreatin has digestive activity only in the much higher pH of an alkaline medium. In contrast, some plant enzymes are stable and active at pH's that can range from 2 through 12. In addition, Infinity2's plant enzymes are optimally active at the temperature of the human body, unlike bromelain and papain.

Secondly, the digestive activity of plant enzymes closely resembles that of food enzymes. They are *not as specific*. These plant enzymes will effectively digest the four main components of food: protein, carbohydrates, fat and fiber. In contrast, pancreatin can break down only three of these four components, while pepsin, trypsin, bromelain and papain can only digest protein.

Thirdly, plant enzymes have *no side effects*, whereas animal enzymes may have some possible side effects. For example, supplying animal enzymes could reduce the human body's ability to create its own enzymes. Pure plant enzymes, on the other hand, do not interfere with the natural functioning of the body and therefore have no side effects.

You might wonder how plant enzymes are prepared.   The Chinese and Japanese originally found that fungi were good producers of acid enzymes and that extracts of various enzymes could be prepared from them. Today, to obtain the desired enzymes, a carefully selected strain of *Aspergillus* is cultured on food materials to which various minerals have been added. Different combinations of various food substrates produce the several enzymes needed such as amylase, proteases, lipase, etc.

The process consists of making a cell fermentation culture using organic whole grain rice (usually) as a nutrient base. The fermentation process produces a rich broth containing the desired enzymes. After fermentation, the enzymes in liquid form are separated completely from all organisms and other nutrients by microfiltration. This broth is filtered five or six times. The result is a very pure protein solution, which is rich in enzymes. This solution is then freeze-dried to produce a stable, concentrated enzyme powder, which is used in **The Enzyme Diet**™.

5.   Glutamine as GlutaMag AAC™.   This particular chelated mineral is noteworthy since it is a very recent innovation in nutritional science. It exploits the important metabolic roles of a rather unique amino acid called glutamine, especially for its role in immune cell activity.

Now, most of the glutamine in the body is stored in skeletal muscle which serves as a source for other body tissues when needed. During strenuous physical activity, illness, injury or nutritional imbalance, plasma levels of glutamine can be reduced and stores depleted at the expense of lean muscle mass. Hence, the value of supplemental glutamine to help maintain lean muscle mass during weight loss.

But glutamine (Glu) itself, as a free amino acid, is not stable in solution and can decompose to form toxic ammonia. The other common alternative in some commercial products is **glutamate** which does **not** contain the extra nitrogen that gives glutamine its special properties. That's where GlutaMagAAC™ becomes the solution.

The key to the stability of glutamine is the bioavailable amino acid chelate (AAC) and the factors that make it nutritionally functional and stable. With GlutaMagAAC™, the research team at Infinity2 has discovered and patented a unique way to stabilize glutamine and thereby include it in **The Enzyme Diet**™ with superior effect in the body.

6.   Essential Fatty Acids. The formulators of **The Enzyme Diet**™ were aware of the important role of essential fatty acids (EFA's) and included both linoleic and linolenic acids. The essential fatty acids are fats that cannot be made by the body, but are required for health, so they must be obtained from food or supplements. When these fatty acids are missing from the diet, symptoms include dry scaly skin, poor wound healing, impaired vision and hearing, fatigue, or liver abnormalities.

There are three essential fatty acids arachidonic acid (AA), linoleic acid (LA) and alpha-linolenic acid (LNA). AA is found primarily in meat and animal products and most people get adequate amounts of this fatty acid. LA is found in pumpkin, sesame and sunflower seeds, walnuts, wheat germ, almonds, pecans and avocados. LNA is found in flax seeds, walnuts and wheat germ. These fatty acids and their ratio in the body play key roles in the proper functioning of cell membranes, hormones, the immune system and are especially important for healthy brain and nerve cells.

Most diets carelessly restrict fats without regard to the level of essential fatty acids. As a result, many dieters are not obtaining adequate amounts of EFA's. To make the problem worse, essential fatty acids are burned at a higher rate when following a calorie-restricted diet. The combination of increased use and a low intake can create a fatty acid deficiency. A fatty acid deficiency can cause fatigue and alter mood, as well as affect the body's ability to build lean muscle, repair tissues, and fight off infection. Therefore, regardless of the type of diet program you're following, you should always make sure that your diet includes adequate amounts of these important fatty acids.

7.   Missing Ingredients.   The health benefits derived from **The Enzyme Diet**™ pertain not only to what it does contain, but also to some conspicuously absent ingredients which are often associated with products like this and which can be harmful or at best, undesirable. As such, it is noteworthy that **The Enzyme Diet**™ is free of ephedra, free of caffeine and in fact free of any other stimulants. It is free of any kind of weight loss **drugs** to suppress appetite, block fat absorption, burn off fat or to do anything else unnatural, like all the quick-fix seekers are looking for. It is also free of lactose so that it is convenient for those who are deficient in the lactase enzyme and do not tolerate this low molecular weight sugar. Speaking of sugar, the product contains less than half the sugar of the average meal replacement shake.

The Enzyme Diet™ *is a product of 15 years of research, six years in development, two years of consumer-testing and now it may be destined to be the number one dietary supplement of choice for effective weight loss everywhere.*

The net effect of this formulation as a meal replacement, when used as part of a healthy lifestyle program, will be to recharge your sluggish metabolism and increase your vitality, while losing the weight you always wanted to, and to enable you to keep it off.

So with all this much to offer, who should use **The Enzyme Diet™?** There's something for everybody.

As a Meal Replacement, The Enzyme Diet™ is ideal because it provides all the nutrients needed to feed the cells; active enzymes and cofactors to maintain metabolism, and an effective delivery system to get them all there. It is therefore **a compelling option** for:

· anyone who would like to lose weight conveniently and effectively, *and*
· anyone who has had difficulty losing weight and keeping it off.

Do you fall into either of these categories? Then pay close attention as you read on into Part III, where you will be able to make the personal application of **The Enzyme Diet™ Solution** just for you.

As a Meal Supplement, The Enzyme Diet™ is an ideal Superfood that provides a rich smorgasbord of essential nutrients, including valuable enzymes and co-factors to aid digestion, absorption and metabolism. Of course, the CAeDS® delivery system will again make it all happen. It is therefore **an attractive option** for:

· anyone who wants the benefits of added nutrition and more importantly, guaranteed cellular nutrition, *and*
· anyone who wants the benefits of increasing his or her intake of valuable supplementary enzymes, quality soy protein, soluble fiber and all the other healthful ingredients.

If you do not have a weight problem, **The Enzyme Diet™** is still good news for you. As a Superfood it will surpass any fast food offering, junk food snack and even a typical American home cooked meal. You can use it as a snack or a meal replacement anytime you choose in your busy schedule. If you have any nutritional concerns at all, this is a choice alternative for you.

৵

Quality Is The Biggest Ingredient

Naturally, when considering any food product, supplement or drug, one must always be concerned about quality. Food products in particular must be preserved for essential freshness and biological activity and at the same time, must be protected from microbiological contamination. Additives can preserve marketability, a practice that is so common in the age of industrial food, but only good natural sources and strict industrial methods and practice can preserve bioavailability.

Your cells know that difference very well. They are not subject to modern media and advertising and are resistant to all sensual appeal. They know nothing but real and essential biological quality. Nothing less will be effective in satisfying their real needs and promoting good health.

The makers of **The Enzyme Diet™** have entered into a strategic alliance with the most prestigious enzyme manufacturing company and has affiliate partnerships with other high-ranking quality manufacturers in the health and nutritional products industry - which manufacture all the ingredients of **The Enzyme Diet™** to maximum standards for quality control and efficacy. This team possesses a unique and proprietary manufacturing component that places their operation above the rest. These partnerships bring unmatched ingenuity and experience to the process.

Skill and commitment to excellence is vitally important in this field because the manufacturing of enzyme-based dietary supplements is a complex operation. There must be a commitment to:

1. Highest quality ingredients and a vendor certification program.
2. Highest quality and state-of-the-art manufacturing processes.
3. Exceptional quality control procedures and the trained specialists to oversee them.

These quality checks include *chromatography* to ensure the quality of all the **ingredients**; *microbiological assays* to ensure **safety**; *enzyme analysis* to ensure maximum **enzyme activity**; *probiotic assays* to ensure a viable **cell count**; and *spectroscopy* to ensure the **bond stability** of the amino acid chelated minerals. Nothing less will do.

Every batch of **The Enzyme Diet™** product undergoes a microbiological contamination analysis. In addition, each raw ingredient is tested for safety, accuracy and quality to ensure that the ingredients are 100% of what the grower claims. Premium products like **The Enzyme Diet**™ go through an average of three times as many quality assurance steps as the law requires and are inspected and tested for quality at every phase of production.

The US FDA now requires that vitamins and other dietary supplements include labels similar to those found on all commercial foods. **Table 5** is a summary of the nutrient information regarding **The Enzyme Diet**™ as it appears on the label.

Table 5 **The Enzyme Diet™ - French Vanilla Flavor**

Nutrition Facts Serving Size: Two scoops. (approx. 35g)

Amount per Serving	with 8 oz water	with skim milk
Calories	123	213
Calories from fat	14	19
	% Daily Value	
Total Fat 2 g	3%	4%
Saturated Fat 0 g	0%	1%
Cholesterol 0 mg	0%	1%
Sodium 136 mg	5%	10%
Total Carbohydrates 14 g	5%	9%
Dietary Fibers 3.7 g	15%	15%

Sugars 6 g

Protein 13 g

Vitamin A 56% • Vitamin C 39% • Calcium 9%
Iron 16% • Magnesium 13% • Zinc 31%
Selenium 133% • Copper 23% • Manganese 140%
Chromium 78% • Molybdenum 124%

When independent laboratories have tested supplements on the market, it was found that some supplements only contain as low as 20% of what is stated on the label. In contrast, independent laboratory tests have shown that **The Enzyme Diet**™ provides 100% or more of what the label claims.

You can have confidence in the quality of **The Enzyme Diet**™. It is the biggest ingredient. There is much more to that than meets the eye and truly, the results and reputation of this innovative diet product lets it speak for itself.

But is there any evidence that it works?

Pilot Studies

Double-blind, randomized clinical trials (RCT's) are almost unheard of when it comes to dieting and weight loss. And there are good reasons for that. This gold standard of the pharmaceutical industry is of utmost importance in protecting patients and the public at large from the potential complications and side effects of therapeutic drugs. Clearly, such RCT's have gone a long way in safeguarding the average consumer from unnecessary morbidity and helped doctors to improve their management of many diseases in modern times.

But in the areas of dieting, supplementation and nutrition in general, it has proven burdensome and often unnecessary to follow the same demanding standards. Here again, **we must avoid the tendency to think in a medical model**. Nutrition is not medicine. These trials are extremely expensive and usually require a long period of time to properly execute them. The verification of the issues involved have not been demanded because of any perceived risks to health per se. The question has been essentially one of efficacy and real benefit. So using the criteria of 'above all, do no harm', there has not been a worrisome threat to create the necessary resolve to carry out this kind of trial. After all, nutrition, especially with natural foods and reasonable protocols, has proven to be eminently safe. There has been truly little to worry about.

Further, because the results we are concerned about are usually multifactoral and the many variables more difficult to control, there has been little commitment (and from just a few quarters) to pursue these types of studies in this general area. In fact, the few significant trials that have been done in recent times have often proven to be contradictory and open to diverse interpretation. Even in the popular media, if you follow the almost weekly accounts of some new observation or development in the area of food nutrients or supplements and their influences on disease prevention or management, you would be most confused in determining what nutritional choices you ought to make.

Think for example, of *The Great Nutrition Debate* that took place in early 2000. That's when some of the nation's best selling diet gurus squared off in a raucous good fight over effective weight loss diet programs. The US Secretary of Agriculture Dan Glickman arranged this national forum, moderated by Carolyn O'Neil of CNN (1). The panelists included Drs. Robert Atkins, Dean Ornish, Barry Sears, Morrison Bethea and John McDougall. They went head to head against each other. The major issue was how to substantiate the long term health impact on dieters of the variety of diet formulas represented among these distinguished doctors. They all had their own formulas that they claim allowed patients to lose weight. No problem there. They acknowledged that across the board, for that's the easy part.

But where were the double blind RCT's to justify any claim to scientific effectiveness in the long run? The few that were brought out caused just as much heated exchange as the obvious lack of unequivocal data. There was so much disagreement over the interpretation of what they each presented. This is dietary warfare, with heat everywhere and not a lot of visible light. *It's no real wonder that many diets used by millions for decades now, have never been subject to randomized clinical trials.* There has hardly been a real need since this is all in the field of nutrition and not medicine. That's the reality. Just think of all the food habits, of all time, used by most people, that have *never been proven.* Why bother?

And yet little or no harm has been done. That's the difference between consuming food and using drugs.

Now, if *they* had such divergence of opinion, and *they* are supposed to be the real experts in this field, imagine the real confusion of the lay person who just wants to lose a few pounds without any hassle or complication and to keep them off.

That's where we are today. Even the best evidence of the best studies to date, leave the best professional experts at loggerheads. Hopefully, as more evidence slowly accumulates and we gain a fuller understanding of the physiology of weight management, the picture will become clearer and decisions such as you would like to make with respect to dietary choices and effective, permanent weight loss, will become much more obvious.

In the meantime, we can report here on three 'pilot' studies that have been concluded to date on **The Enzyme Diet™**. The results are consistently positive.

A User Survey - Samples of **The Enzyme Diet™** were provided to about 50 typical consumers to try. These customers reported back on taste, weight loss results and overall general comments about the product. All of these customers lost weight using the product, but not all of them liked the taste, etc. Adjustments to the flavor and formula were made, based on their feedback. This survey was very informal and there was no control for other dietary and lifestyle factors such as exercise, diet, medications, etc. The weight loss during the four months of the survey varied from one pound per week to as much as ten pounds in one week. Some of the more obese individuals lost very large amounts of weight, especially in the first few weeks of using the product. Because this was a very informal survey and numerous variables were not controlled, the resulting information would not meet 'scientific' criteria for demonstrable validity. But it was all positive.

A Small Preliminary Study.

- A group of five healthy women between the ages of 25 and 40 were placed on the pilot version of **The Enzyme Diet™** for eight weeks. Body fat, weight, girth measurements and resting metabolic rate were measured. Resting metabolic rate was measured using a gas-exchange system from MedGraphics. Measurements were taken at baseline, four weeks and eight weeks. The average fat loss (calculated through body fat measurements using skinfold calipers) for this group was 1.75 pounds per week and none of the women experienced a drop in metabolic rate during the study. Again, due to the small number of subjects, even though there was more rigorous monitoring of them, these results were not sufficiently thorough or statistically weighted to be publishable after peer review. Nevertheless, the results are just what you would expect from our current state of knowledge.

Consumer-testing A pilot version of **The Enzyme Diet**™ was released for use by Infinity2 customers and health practitioners. Informal feedback from the health practitioners and customers about the success of the product was obtained. There is a return policy that allows individuals who are not satisfied with the product for any reason to return the product for a refund. During the two years of testing, there was less than a 1% return rate (the actual return rate was 3 of 1,000 participants or 0.3%). There were many scattered reports from customers and health practitioners about individual success in using **The Enzyme Diet**™ to keep the weight off. Those who have continued to use **The Enzyme Diet**™ regularly have been able to keep the weight off. Those who stopped using the product and stopped following a healthy diet (i.e. returning to pizza and burgers, etc), gained some weight back, but did not necessarily gain back all the weight or return to their pre-diet weight. Again, all these results to date have been very positive and encouraging.

At some time in the future, it may be possible to perform an 'official scientific multi-center clinical' of **The Enzyme Diet**™. However, in the meantime, thousands are already discovering that it works.

◊

The Enzyme Diet™ WORKS!

The Enzyme Diet™ uses the power of enzymes to support your metabolism at its optimum level without drugs or stimulants. Your body will burn the maximum amount of fat by pulling your excess fat from storage by normal enzyme action and using it as fuel. You need not go through the usual starvation mode and there should be little or no slowing of your metabolism. You will lose mostly fat and not cannibalize your lean muscle. In effect, your body will get a kind of "metabolic makeover". It works!

It has been most exciting to observe the results that people have received using **The Enzyme Diet™** and the positive changes it has brought in their lives. Below are a few exemplary stories from among the thousands of individuals who have had great success using this simple approach to help them achieve their weight loss and health goals. They tell it in their own words:

Jill M. Longwood, FL
(Female, 57, Lost 95 lbs,)   **"Saved my life"**

"The Enzyme Diet™ has saved my life. I have now lost 95 pounds and I can't tell you what a dramatic difference this product has made in my life. I have always had a weight problem. I was very tired, depressed, despondent, and had neither energy nor desire to do anything.

"When I started on The Enzyme Diet™ I weighed 257 pounds. In the second week the pounds started falling off. I started feeling better. I started having more energy. I started getting excited.

"I have now lost an astounding 95 pounds. I have gone from 257 to 162 in 9 months. I am totally a new person. I have energy like I haven't had in years. My doctor is now ordering the product for her husband.

"I have a new life. I feel young again. I am now a new person. I feel great. I now want to look my best again. The Enzyme Diet™ has truly been a solution to my weight and health problems. It has given me a new life!"

Ron M., Longwood, FL
(Male, 53, Lost 80 lbs)　　　　**"Words cannot describe"**

"The Enzyme Diet™ is fantastic! Discovering this product has truly been a life changing experience. I have found new youth. I set a ridiculous goal to lose 82 pounds when I started on this product. This would get me down to one pound less than I weighed when my wife and I got married. Incredibly, I've now lost 80 pounds, from 266 to 186, in 10 months with The Enzyme Diet™. Words cannot describe what this product has done for me. I have energy that I haven't had since my twenties. I feel great. The Enzyme Diet™ has completely changed my life."

Judy L., Vancouver, WA
(Female, 63, Lost 57 lbs)　　　**"The weight loss has been so fast"**

"Jim and I have been overweight since day one of our 43 years of wedded bliss. Due to some health problems that we both have, it was decided that we would commit ourselves to starting "another" diet.

"I was a heavy meat and fat eater and low calorie diets had never worked for me in the past as I was always starved for and craved meat and foods that were high in fat. Therefore, I was not looking forward to the craving that I felt would take place with this 'new diet product.' Jim and I have been on the diet continuously since our starting date. I can't believe this product. We are losing weight regularly and at a fast pace, but most importantly, I do not have the craving that I had on all the other diets. As of this date, Jim has lost 37 lbs and I have lost 57 lbs. Even though we gained some weight while on a week's vacation, we not only lost that but more by the first week home and back on schedule. We have energy that we have never had before. There have also been some side benefits that we never even dreamed of.

"Our friends can't get over how we look and that the weight loss has been so fast. Most men carry their fat in their tummy, not their butt, thighs and legs. All a man has to do is lose 2 ounces and everyone notices his weight loss. This is a man thing. A woman has fat in every cell of her body and it takes weeks before anyone notices she is losing weight. This diet has been different in that area as well. People began noticing the weight loss and loss of inches within 2 weeks. That never happened when we were on other diets as it always took three to four weeks. After we reach our goal, we will continue to use this fantastic product. I can see where the weight loss will be easy to maintain.

"Another big thing about this diet with me is the taste. I love The Enzyme Diet™ drink! I can't wait to get up in the morning and get my first drink of it. This may sound dumb, but taste really does play a big part when dieting. You have two customers for life from this family."

Joan H., Ken H., Medicine Hat, AB
(Female, 55, Lost 49 lbs, Male, 58, Lost 28 lbs)"Bought ... new clothes"

"We both started on TED and in a short period of time, Joan has lost 35 lbs. and I lost 21 lbs. As of today, we are down 49 and 26 pounds respectively. I had to put five new notches in my belt and went from wearing size 41 to 38 pants. Joan just went out and bought some new clothes because the old ones she dug out of the closet were just too baggy. We like what TED is doing for our energy level. Thanks!"

John R., Maple Grove, MN
(Male, 50, Lost 100 lbs)   "My quality of life increased 10-fold"

"When I was first introduced to The Enzyme Diet™ I was skeptical. I was extremely obese and had been on many diets in the past that didn't work for me. Due to the money back guarantee, I decided to try it anyway. I felt I had nothing to lose. In the first few days of being on the diet, I could feel something was going on with my body. I definitely had increased energy and just generally felt better.

"I started thinking about weighing myself, something I hadn't done in a couple of years. The problem was finding a scale to use. I tried my doctor's office, my chiropractor's office, and the local clinic. I couldn't find a scale that would weigh anything over 350lbs. I was discouraged, but because of the way the diet was making me feel, I had to figure out something. I finally ended up sneaking into my company's shipping department and used their freight scale. When I finally saw what I weighed, I checked it 3 times. I knew from the other scales that I was over 350, but I really found it hard to believe I weighed in at 382 lbs!

"In thinking back, I shouldn't have been that surprised. I had just bought a pair of pants with a 58-inch waist, I have a job sitting at a desk all day, and it's hard for me to exercise due to a hip that needs to be replaced. That was 8 months ago. I have followed the diet as much as possible since. Only weighing myself once a week for months out of necessity, I started seeing the pounds come off. My pants started getting baggy and I could do a lot more without having to stop and catch my

breath. *My quality of life increased 10 fold.*

"I am forever grateful for The Enzyme Diet™. It has changed my life! I haven't had to use the freight scale in months. I have more energy than I've had in years! I am now able to wear 46-inch pants, and I currently am weighing in at 282 lbs. That brings my total pounds lost to 100!"

Judy H., Buda, TX
(Female, 49, Lost 65 lbs)   **"My doctor was so surprised"**

"After one particular very bad day, I decided to make a list of everything, within my control, that was making me unhappy, and make changes. At the top of my list was my weight. I had tried pills, liquid diets, and almost every other method trying to lose weight. I had never found a program, which I could stick with and that worked with no side effects.

"One day, my sister told me about The Enzyme Diet™ (TED), which she was trying along with her co-workers. I started TED at a weight of 237 pounds. To my delight, the weight immediately started falling off and I wasn't hungry. As of this writing, I have lost 65 pounds. I plan to lose 100 pounds- my goal!

"I feel great! After losing 49 pounds, I had my annual physical, and it was the best physical I've had in years. My doctor was so surprised that my cholesterol and triglycerides were down. TED is incredibly easy to follow and stick to. Before TED, I always skipped breakfast because I didn't have time and didn't like to eat early in the day. TED has solved that problem because it's so quick, easy, and delicious! Now, I never skip meals. I have a shake for breakfast and dinner on most days and eat sensibly at lunch. I have fruit for snacks.

"After 6 months on the program, I am still very motivated. I was born with a weak digestive tract and have been on medication for it most of my life. TED is very soothing to my stomach, and I rarely suffer from nausea anymore. I noticed, immediately, that I had more energy. The more pounds I lost, the more the energy increased. I felt so much younger that I made a game out of it. I told my friend, Marilyn, that I had a new boyfriend named 'TED' and that we were on a Birthday Diet. Since my beginning weight was 237, I pretended to be 23. I was a bit skeptical at first, but when my weight dropped below 200 pounds and I was a teenager again (19 when I hit 199 pounds), I called and left a message on my

friend's voice mail and sang Happy Birthday to myself. Before I knew it, I was 18 and feeling like it, too. Now I'm only 17, going on 16, and I'm making plans for my first cruise! I have 5 grandchildren, and the younger ones are so lucky to have a Grandma with a lap. I am able to do so many things now that I couldn't do before because of lack of energy, mobility, or both. I am extremely happy, feel healthier, and TED has given me my life back."

Ruby C., Charlotte, NC
(Female, 67, Lost 31 lbs)　　"Great to wear short sleeves again"

"Today will be 132 days on TED. I have lost 31 pounds. I've never been able to lose the 'fat' on my upper arms until now. It's great to wear short sleeves again! I have gone from a very tight 16 petite to size 12 petite. I've lost numerous pains in my body, and my self-esteem is at an all time high. The blouse I have on is 32 years old - one of my favorites - but I never could wear it because of fat arms! I do want to lose another 20-25 pounds. I know that TED and I can do it."

Bob C., Dover, FL
(Male, 44, Lost 55 lbs)　　　"Nothing can stop me now"

"Without a doubt, The Enzyme Diet™ has dramatically changed my life. Other people can't imagine what it is like to weigh 400 pounds. There are so many things you can't do. You try to stay away from things that involve any activity. You can only live half a life.

"My family has always been in the food business in New Jersey. Following the family tradition, I've owned restaurants, delis, and now I own a catering and lunch-truck business here in Florida. We have to start the day around 4:00 in the morning to prepare the food and have the trucks loaded for our breakfast routes. I used to stuff weenie wraps and chicken fingers in my mouth first thing in the morning before 5A.M. Then I would eat non-stop through the rest of the day.

"The obese life is a slowed down life. You physically can't do what other people can do, and your health really suffers. My calves were so tight with edema and poor circulation that I couldn't stand it. Now I've lost 2 ½" in each calf and my body is so much more comfortable. Because of being overweight, I had sleep apnea. I've had 15 different accidents where I ran off the road because I fell asleep. Once I took out the gate at Rooms To Go. All the security guards surrounded the truck. I

didn't even know what happened. I'm lucky I never hurt anybody. Because of the weight loss I don't have sleep apnea anymore.

"Before I was introduced to The Enzyme Diet™ in August I had struggled to get my weight down from 408 to 383. When I tried The Enzyme Diet™, I immediately knew something was different. I had been out of control for so long that when I felt the control of my appetite and the control of my food intake, I knew this time things were really going to be different! There was a change in me from the very beginning. I had no problem doing the shake from day one. It tastes good and it is easy. I feel physically stronger, more energetic, and I am more mentally alert. "In just under 3 months, I've taken off another 55 pounds for a total of 80. I now weigh 328. Besides the weight loss on The Enzyme Diet™, I have now lost 50 inches over my entire body. I am looking forward to playing sports again. I used to play basketball and softball. By next spring I think I will be down enough to join some sports teams. At least I know I will have the energy to play! Another thing I have wanted to do was expand my business. I used to be so tired that I never felt like it was the right time to do it. Now I have plenty of energy, more confidence and a really positive outlook on life. I am ready to take on that challenge now.

"The Enzyme Diet™ has given me my life back. The nurse who shared it with me says, 'I'm a heat-seeking missile.' I am locked in on my target weight and nothing can stop me now!"

Stephen T., Riverside, CA
(Male, 51, Lost 32 lbs)   **"Changing lives for the better"**
"I started using The Enzyme Diet™ plan and knew immediately that this was it for me. It tasted great and it did what it stated it would do. It gave me that filled feeling, and yet I knew I was getting all the nutrients I needed for my day. I have lost a total of 33 lbs. and it feels great. I have more energy at home and at work and all my co-workers want to know what has happened to me. I tell them about The Enzyme Diet™ plan and I now have a dozen people using this product at my workplace! I feel great about being a part of changing lives for the better."

Grace B., Bermuda
(Female, 61, Lost 35lbs)   **"The answer to my prayers"**
"While doing some housekeeping chores at the home of my

youngest son, as his wife was abroad, I barely had enough energy to complete three hours in a 2 level house. I felt badly, because I had run my own Maid Service and Cleaning Company, and sometimes while training I always considered myself fast and thorough.

"*My first reaction to The Enzyme Diet™ was that I received so much energy. And now 5 ½ months later it is incredible the energy I have. I previously weighed 200 pounds. Now my weight has come down to 165. I am happy to report that I have lost 6 inches off my waist - from 42 to 36. My dress size has gone from a woman's 16 to a misses 14. The Enzyme Diet™ has been the answer to my prayers.*"

Chris K., Zirconia, NC
(Male, 30, Lost 15lbs)   "Saves me time and money"
"*I gained some unwanted pounds in the course of this last spring and summer while attending college, especially this last summer. There was no canteen or grill open on campus and all of my classes were so close together that I did not have time to go off campus for lunch. I ended up eating junk food out of the snack machines and drinking sodas a lot. In the meantime, I was not getting much exercise either. So several pounds were added to my weight.*

"*I ordered T.E.D. and let it sit on the shelf, but eventually got serious about losing weight and put it to the test. I was not disappointed! I lost 10 pounds in the first 5 days of using the product! I then went on a mini-vacation with my wife and gained a couple of pounds from overeating. When I returned home, I went back on T.E.D. and lost another 5 pounds in a matter of days! It tastes great, is convenient, easy to use, and saves me time and money! Thank you for this phenomenal product.*"

Penny B, Hudson, NH
(Female, Lost 24lbs)   "I feel great"
"*I'm a stay at home mom. I have been looking for a solution to my weight problem since my kids were babies, and since being on The Enzyme Diet™ I feel great. I have tons of energy and it only took 10 weeks to lose 24 pounds, 11inches and to buy some new summer clothes 2 dress sizes smaller.*"

Mel __., Corpus Christie, TX
(Male, 80, Lost 35 lbs)   **"I feel great" at 80!**

"I'm 80 years old. I've been on The Enzyme Diet™ for 3 months I've lost 35 pounds. As a result of my weight loss my blood pressure had dropped at least 20 points I feel great."

Don B., Longwood, FL
(Male, 50 lbs)   **"Amazing Transformations"**

"Since starting The Enzyme Diet™ in February, amazing transformations have occurred. In the first 21 days, I went from 410 pounds to 380 pounds - 30lbs. I have to use 2 scales to weigh. Normally when I use my wife's Saturn, I have to move the seat back all the way, and tilt it back one notch. Last Thursday I just got in the car. The fit was a little tight, but it was in my wife's position, not mine. I was then able to reach down and adjust the seat back, but no tilting of the seat back. My gut didn't touch the steering wheel. While helping my wife (who has lost 20lbs too) put up a ceiling fan, my pants dropped to my ankles. Friday night I walked from our auto repair shop to my home, about ¼ of a mile. My hip joints will normally burn - but not this time. The same thing was true when I went to get the car the next day. My total weight loss goal is to be at 180lbs - that's another 200lbs. With The Enzyme Diet™ I can now feel this goal is attainable and that I will be able to keep it off for life. I hope to keep you up to date as time progresses."

☙

Questions & Answers

1. Can I prepare The Enzyme Diet™ ahead of time and keep it refrigerated?

Preparing **The Enzyme Diet™** and storing it in the refrigerator for more than 20 minutes is not recommended, as this deactivates some of the vital enzymes. You will experience the best results by preparing it according to the package directions and drinking it right away. (Two scoops mixed with 8 ounces of cold water or skim milk). Shaking rather than stirring the mixture will result in a smoother, thicker drink.

2. I feel more energy after taking The Enzyme Diet™; is this common?

Most people report that their energy levels are higher after drinking The Enzyme Diet™. Some people even experience a mild "rush" of energy. There are no drugs or stimulants - the effects you are feeling may be the result of it boosting your body's metabolic systems into "full production" mode, thereby giving you more energy.

3. How long can I stay on The Enzyme Diet™ weight-loss program?

As long as you desire. Because it is highly nutritious and completely natural, it may actually improve your nutritional status. Once you have achieved your desired weight, you can continue drinking a serving each day as a meal replacement as part of your new healthy lifestyle.

4. Can I use The Enzyme Diet™ if I am pregnant, lactating or have a medical condition?

It contains only all-natural, whole food nutrients, but with your condition, you should talk with your health professional before beginning any diet or exercise program.

5. I have been taking The Enzyme Diet™ for a few days and feel very hungry ... is this normal?

If you are a chronic dieter or have quite a bit of weight to lose, it is likely that your metabolism has already been slowed dramatically. With The Enzyme Diet™, your metabolism becomes more active than it is used to, and you may feel extremely hungry at first. If this happens, drink an extra serving to satisfy your appetite. And don't worry, as your metabolism resets itself, this intense hunger should subside.

6. I have been taking The Enzyme Diet™ for two days and feel tired and sluggish. Is this normal?

A small number of people may feel tired or sluggish when they first start taking it, as their bodies undergo metabolic changes. It fires up the body's metabolic systems, which may make you feel worse before better. Any negative feelings should subside in a few days, so just keep following the program and you will be well on your way to looking and feeling better than you ever have.

7. What makes The Enzyme Diet™ unique?

It is the only meal replacement product that contains:
i. Key Enzymes to help maintain your metabolism as you lose weight.
ii. All the Essential natural-source nutrients to feed your cells, and
iii. An Effective delivery system to get them there.

8. Is The Enzyme Diet™ FDA approved?

The FDA only grants 'approvals' on substances considered to be drugs. Therefore, the FDA approval process is not applicable to all-natural products like The Enzyme Diet™.

9. Are there any known drug interactions with The Enzyme Diet™? Do I have to change any of my medications?

No. As a food product, there are no obvious contraindications and no interactions with any therapeutic drugs have ever been observed or reported. However, if your medication states explicitly that it should be taken 'on an empty stomach', you should not take that medication at the same time as The Enzyme Diet™, since it is considered a food. If you have any anxiety or concern, be sure to consult with your personal physician.

10. How does The Enzyme Diet™ compare with other meal replacements on the market today?

The answer to this loaded question can perhaps be best summarized in **Table 6** on the next page. The comparison is then self-explanatory.

Table 6   **A Comparison of Meal Replacements**

Drink	Calories	Fat Grams	Sugar Grams	Contains Enzymes?	Contains Chelated Minerals?	Contains Soy Protein for Heart Health?	Contains a Nutrient Delivery System
The Enzyme Diet™	123	2	6	Y	Y	Y	Y
Slim Fast Regular - Ready to drink can	220	3	35	N	N	N	N
Soy - Ready to drink can	170	2	12	N	N	Y	N
SlimFast Ultra Soy-chocolate powder	170	2	12	N	N	Y	N
Metabolite	220	3	35	N	N	N	N
Boost	240	4	27	N	N	N	N
Ensure Plus	360	11	16	N	N	N	N
Ensure Light	200	3	18	N	N	N	N
Appeal Lite (Nu Skin)	210	2	26	N	N	N	N
Instant Breakfast	220	0	34	N	N	N	N
Sweet Success	200	3	30	N	N	N	N
Small McDonalds Shake*	360	9	55	N	N	N	N
12oz Can of Coke*	140	0	39	N	N	N	N

* Although a McDonald's shake and a 12 oz coke are not meal replacements, they are included as a comparison to demonstrate the high fat and sugar content of many meal replacement shakes.

Part III

ଓଃ

Your Personal
APPLICATION

Are You Framing A Winning Plan?

❧ *Chapter 7* ❧

DEVELOP YOUR PLAN
Lose Weight, Not Control.

Now, there's hope! There is a *solution* to the *problem* of continuous, ineffective yo-yo dieting.

It's time to move on to your personal *application*. In Part I we discussed the real need to address the silent, growing epidemic in America because of the health implications of overweight and obesity. So many popular diets remain an elusive remedy because they fail to address the real crux of the problem. However, from Part II you now have a new awareness of the role of enzymes in human metabolism and the need for adequate nutrition to feed your cells, plus a delivery system to maximize those dietary benefits. An innovative approach has been developed which you now know as **The Enzyme Diet™** -- the meal replacement with a winning difference. But that's not the whole story. **The Enzyme Diet™ Solution** is a comprehensive program to afford you effective weight loss that stays lost.

The Enzyme Diet™ supports the body's metabolic enzyme systems allowing it to burn a maximum amount of energy, while consuming only a relatively small amount of calories - all without the usual cravings or hunger. These enzymes require specific nutrients (vitamins, minerals, amino acids, etc.) to function properly. Most low calorie diets don't provide enough of all these nutrients and the result is loss of lean body mass, reduced metabolism and post diet weight gain.

The Enzyme Diet™ includes all the necessary nutrients to support the body's metabolic enzymes. It also provides the digestive enzymes necessary to ensure that those nutrients are absorbed and delivered to the cells with maximum efficiency. The result is safe and efficient weight loss, increased energy and overall improved health - with no drugs, stimulants or synthetic ingredients.

Do you need to lose weight? That's the basic question you obviously need to answer for yourself before you even attempt to develop a personal Application of **The Enzyme Diet™ Solution**. We know there are potential health consequences for individuals who have a BMI >25 and especially for those who are clinically obese with a BMI >30. The answer for you if you fall into either category is obvious. For health reasons alone, you should definitely seek to reduce your weight.

Or perhaps, it's a matter of self image. You would look better and feel better if you had a few less pounds to carry around. It matters to you, even though you have a healthy body image, with no illusions to prompt any kind of eating disorders. It's your preference and a priority now on your agenda. You want to do something about it. You may even have tried before, but now you understand what you need to do.

So how do you apply this innovative meal replacement alternative to your personal situation? How can you take advantage of all these proven benefits to address your weight challenge? Can you avoid the common dieting mistakes that so many millions continue to make as they try to solve their problems, only to end up with disgusting failure and frustration? As you seek to develop your own effective weight loss program, you want to avoid these negative pitfalls and devise a plan that will result in your personal success.

Let's first review *The Success Cycle*.

THE SUCCESS CYCLE

In one of my previous books *A Passion for Living*, (Gunnars and Campbell, 1993) I developed a simple universal paradigm which I called *The Success Cycle* illustrated on the next page (Fig. 1). It is a convenient representation of the **TEN STEPS** necessary for anyone to achieve almost anything worthwhile. Effective weight loss is no exception. Let me explain.

Step One of the Success Cycle illustrates that all your personal achievement must begin with taking *personal responsibility* or ownership of your endeavor. You look inside for the reserve and take initiative toward change and success. You stop blaming anyone or anything else. You stop waiting for some moving train. You fire your own engines. **Step Two** identifies the *desire* you must tap into to have, to do or to be whatever you choose for yourself. It is a fountain of energy springing up inside that constrains you to act, to change and to grow. You do it all because you really want to. **Step Three** demands a specific focus or *goal* that intensifies your desire like a magnifying glass focuses the rays of the sun to create a burning heat. You become motivated with electricity and that makes you so magnetic that you begin to attract everything you need to fulfil your ultimate goal. That goal makes you electro-magnetic.

Fig. 1

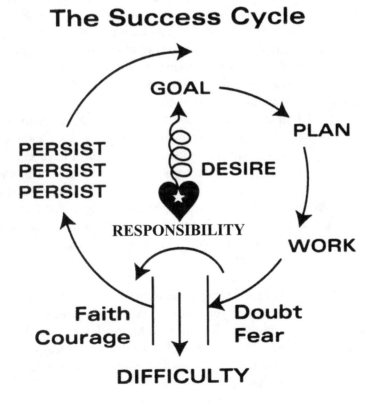

The Success Cycle

GOAL

PLAN

PERSIST
PERSIST
PERSIST

DESIRE

RESPONSIBILITY

WORK

Faith
Courage

Doubt
Fear

DIFFICULTY

But you must then develop a step-wise *plan* in **Step Four**. This breaks down the daunting challenge of any proportion, into a series of small manageable steps that begin at your feet, wherever you are right now. Your plan allows you to pace yourself and measure your progress. Then you go to *work* in **Step Five**. Nothing worth having, doing or being will ever come easy. But you learn to work smart and not necessarily hard. You always use your brain before your body. And you practice brainstorming with the mastermind principle to gain maximum efficiency in everything you do.

Inevitably you will encounter *difficulty* in **Step Six**. Nothing comes free and nothing comes easy. It is through opposition and struggle that you develop strength and stamina. It is by your worst mistakes that you learn your most important lessons. It is through the path of failure that you cultivate success. But you must learn the lessons. Your first response in **Step Seven** is always to *doubt* yourself - can you do it? You doubt your mission - is it worth it? You doubt the future - is it possible? And you are prone to *fear*. You become afraid of failure, afraid of embarrassment, afraid of imaginary creations of your own mind. Such doubt and fear are emotions that threaten to take you out of the game. They siphon off losers from the cycle of success.

Step Eight calls for you to overcome this tendency to freeze - paralyzed by doubt and fear. It summons you to make a conscious choice in the face of your present difficulty. You choose to have *faith*. You choose to believe that you can succeed. You affirm that your mission or your goal is worth it. You redefine your future as you determine it to be. Faith then replaces doubt. Similarly, you take *courage*. You find the will to overcome your fear by attacking it head on. You make the big decision. You'll do it, no matter what. You jump in - hook, line and sinker. You pass the point of no return.

The rest is then a breeze. You can now *persist* and *persist* and *persist*. You hang in there in **Step Nine** until the inevitable happens. You would never quit just before you realize your goal. You see it coming and like a marathoner around the last curve in the road, who can see the finish line up ahead, even if your stomach aches, and your feet wobble and your lungs well nigh collapse, you find miraculous reserve to finish because your goal summons you irresistibly.

But you are not content to retire just yet. You know that if you are not careful, you will go around in the same circle as before. That will carve a hole and you'll fall into a rut. That rut threatens to become a trench and if you fall into it, it will become your grave. So you redefine a new goal in **Step Ten** which changes the circle into a *spiral* of success. Now each time you go around, you find the process is unending and real retirement comes only at the end of life. Your life itself becomes an expanding and exhilarating challenge that takes you past each horizon into new worlds of experience that you never imagined possible.

That is *The Success Cycle*. It is a universal paradigm that exposes the anatomy of how things happen by human achievement or alternately why results do not always follow the best of human intentions. Weight loss is no exception.

∾

Common Dieting Mistakes

Now, let's look at the ten common dieting mistakes which can be labeled at each of these Ten Steps that we have just described.

Mistake #1. If You Fail To TAKE RESPONSIBILITY.

You deny your weight problem is **your** problem. It's not your fault at all. It was because your mom fed you too much as a baby. Or your hormones make you fat. It's your bad luck. You only watch food and you gain weight. It's in your genes, you're programmed that way.

But you really do know, especially since you've got this far in this book, that you must somehow deal with the *energy (calorie) balance equation*. You can and do make lifestyle choices that influence your weight one way or the other. So the prayer of St. Francis comes back to haunt you. Sure, you must have the patience to accept what you truly cannot change. But you must also have the courage to change what can be changed and best of all, you must have the wisdom to know that difference. It's your game and only yours. The Solution to your weight issue is in your hands. Alone!

Mistake #2. If You Really Have No DESIRE For Change

Trying to lose weight without having a clear idea of how it will benefit you, is a complete waste of time. If you are not motivated from within, you'll be facing a losing battle, for sure. This is something you must really want to do. You should do it for nobody but yourself. It's really a personal kind of thing. You must make the decision and no one else.

In the extreme, you may even get to the point where you don't care anymore. You just don't care. Let everybody else be concerned about your weight, but it just won't bother you. That would be just fine, if all you have to lose is just a few pounds in the wrong places. There are really no other consequences. But if you are truly overweight or even obese, that choice is really not yours to make. At least not without implications for your health. Therefore, in such a situation, you are almost obliged to take action. Your physician now has something to suggest - more than suggest - to prescribe. Just a word to the wise should usually be sufficient.

If you have the desire, you'll take control. You will make a definite choice to alter your lifestyle. You'll choose a sensible weight loss plan like **The Enzyme Diet™ Solution**. You'll alter your eating habits completely. You'll start to exercise. You won't allow people or situations to drive your impulses. You'll pause before you react. That way, you won't take out your stress and frustration on food. You'll be in the driver's seat with appropriate stress management and alternate conflict resolution. You'll deal with your own anger, frustrations, inferiority complex, boredom or whatever emotion constrains you to go on a binge. All because you want to. Your desire will dictate your new disciplined lifestyle. Your weight loss will become your thing.

Mistake #3. If You Set Unrealistic Expectations or GOALS

You've seen the ads, you've heard the claims. You've looked at the models and even some of your friends, and then you looked in the mirror. So you decided that you were going to become somebody else. You were going to lose all the weight that you did not want anymore. You'd drop five or six sizes in clothes. You'd perhaps lose 30 or even 40% of your weight, if you thought you really were obese. Or, on the other extreme, you border on being anorexic. Well, not quite, but you insist on losing that extra five or ten pounds, no matter what. Nobody else knows but you, '*how fat*' you are. You have images of a slimmer, trimmer, fitter you that you must realize.

Both extremes would be a big mistake. You will frustrate yourself if you focus on being half your size or something as ridiculous as that, at the outset. Similarly, you would always be dissatisfied if you harbor a distorted sense of your own body image, thinking that losing just the few extra pounds you detest will transform your visual appearance.

It really is important that you have a realistic goal that does justice to your present height and weight, to your personal history, your age, your health status and your lifestyle. As a rule of thumb, you would always be wise to set as an initial goal to lose no more than ten percent of your pre-dieting weight. This is almost certainly achievable by a sensible weight loss program like **The Enzyme Diet™Solution.** It defines a clear and adequate starting point and best of all, studies show that all the health consequences of excess weight begin to be reversed by this simple quantitative change. It is possible and it is beneficial ... therefore, it's worth it. You simply need to have patience. It will take time to do it right. Imagine yourself 10% reduced all round. Your self image will improve immediately and you will begin to feel the benefit even as you start out on your new program.

Mistake #4.   If You Fail to Develop A PLAN

You decide you need to lose some weight. That's good. So you just go on some diet that allows you to eat less. You cut back on all the foods you know are 'fattening.' Or, you just begin to follow some diet you find in a popular diet book. Or, you add some pill that is supposed to cut your appetite or 'burn fat' in some way. Or, you join some group that has you fall in line in a restrictive program of some kind. You have no real plan of your own. You do not know your daily routines or responsibilities and you have no way to monitor or evaluate your progress. So you drift aimlessly and hopelessly, responding to impulse and suggestions from every quarter. You get nowhere.

Surely, you need to have a definitive plan. This should include a starting date, a daily schedule or routine and a step wise goal. To lose say two or three pounds per week *after* your first week would be almost ideal for most people. Your plan might include strict disciplines you impose to control your impulse behavior. You may have fixed arrangements for shopping for food, for eating out and for exercise and fluid intake. You might keep a diary record of your diet, exercise and weight, to monitor your progress. And how about holding yourself accountable, to yourself for sure, or maybe to your spouse, your children, a friend? These are the kinds of things you must determine in an organized program for success in dieting and effective weight loss. You will need also an exit strategy and a maintenance program. If you put this all together, you'll take the guesswork out of your endeavor. You'll know exactly what you're about and how to apply necessary checks and balances. Aim to lose weight and keep it off, not by default but by design.

Mistake #5.   If You Fail To WORK At It.

You think that (somehow) you'll just start losing weight automatically. You make no effort to learn about your body or your behavior. You do not learn what constitutes healthy eating or what benefits are to be derived from a moderate exercise program. Speaking of exercise, you continue in a sedentary lifestyle. You spend hours in front of the TV or use every means of transportation at your disposal. You sleep in on weekends. Not much changes, except for skipping meals or avoidance of all those big steaks and sweet desserts you once enjoyed. And yet you keep stepping on the scale in hopes of seeing the needle shift to the left. Recall that definition of *insanity* about doing the same things and yet expecting different results.

Working at weight loss involves three indispensable work components. First, you must do your *homework.* That involves reading, learning, seeking out all the reliable information you can find about the essential principles of effective dieting. Hopefully you've learned a lot already from this book. You need to understand the nature of food and what is adequate, balanced nutrition. You need to learn of lifestyle consequences. Secondly, you need to *work out.* Get into an exercise program or routine such as you'll discover in a later chapter. Be consistent at it, for it will pay off. Thirdly, *work on yourself* - your mental gymnastics. Cultivate a healthy, positive self image. Exercise the discipline and self control to follow your plan. If the going gets tough, be tough and keep going.

Mistake #6.   If You Are Surprised By DIFFICULTY.

Dieting is not easy. Losing weight is not easy. That's obvious from all the data and reports that clearly show the vast majority of people who try to lose weight, either fail in their early attempts, or they succeed to some degree in the short term, and then are disappointed later to watch the scales creep back up, sometimes even above where they started. This has been a difficult proposition across the board. Don't be surprised if you hit an early plateau. All dieters, have 'bad days.' Don't be surprised if you lose the battle in any given week.

When you apply **The Enzyme Diet™ Solution**, the difficulty will not be with the scales. You will find that if you follow a good program, you will lose weight and you will not suffer the cravings and hunger pangs that haunt many a dieter on most other weight loss programs. You will not be prone to continue the yo-yo pattern that frustrates the typical person who loses weight in the short-term and then fails to keep it off in the medium to long term. That's not where your difficulty will lie. Rather, the difficulty will be to affirm your healthy self image and to maintain the discipline to pursue real behavior modification.

You will have to avoid the emotional crises that lead to impulsive eating, and follow your consistent exercise program. When you have a bad day, you should sometimes just go with the flow, enjoy the binge for what it is worth, but then immediately get back on your diet program. Don't be too hard on yourself. That way you'll only delay your weight loss just a bit. Change makes its own demands and you must be prepared to cope with its consequences. Difficulty will either make you stronger and therefore lighter in weight, or it will cause you to give up and to watch your weight creep up by neglect or default.

Mistake #7. If You Give In To DOUBT and FEAR

These are normal, spontaneous and emotional reactions to difficulty when it does come - in whatever form. You may have tried to lose weight before - maybe just once or perhaps several times. But when your weight stagnates or oscillates, or you just can't seem to get past some wall of opposition - then it is easy to doubt that you'll ever weigh less than you do. You will never look better and you will never feel better. You doubt that it is worth the effort at all. You doubt that it even matters and you could even cease to care any more.

You go a step further. Emotions take over. You shrink in fear. What an overwhelming sense that could be. To be afraid of inevitable failure is to condemn yourself to a prison of paralysis. You imagine not just being what you are but even getting worse. You fear you could even be fat, or more fat. You fear the consequences. You fear you could collapse if you exercise. Your self image collapses. You withdraw. You're prone to depression and ultimate defeat.

What a negative cycle to be in. That's a hopeless state, unless you choose a different one.

Mistake #8. If You Do Not Choose To BELIEVE and Do Not Have The COURAGE to Act

In such negative circumstances you always have a choice to make. You can choose to believe. You choose to see yourself as the person you really want to be. Not an exaggerated or unrealistic stereotype. But rather, you choose to reconstruct a mental picture of limited change. Just a few less pounds. Just a bit smaller, thinner, trimmer. You insist that must be possible. You affirm all you know about the *energy (calorie) balance equation* and the fundamentals of physiology. If you do the right thing, you will inevitably get the right result. So you are willing to try and to keep trying. You put your foot down. You gain the courage to act. You're soon back on the program. Anxiety now gives way to confidence. Despair now turns to hope. Depression slowly transforms into joy.

Mistake #9. If You Give Up And Not PERSIST.

You lose! You don't lose weight. You lose life as it could be, or might have been! You never become the person you really wanted to be!

Life is facing challenge, if it is anything. It is a journey and not a destination, a struggle and not a victory. So, choose to live!

Mistake #10. If You Do Not Make Permanent LIFESTYLE CHANGE

An effective weight loss program is not an interval of time wherein you follow some imposed restrictions to lose a few pounds. It is a way of life. Your goal is to lose weight and to keep it off. What you do to lose it is synonymous with what you do to keep it off. The lifestyle change must be permanent. You change your dietary habits for life. No more empty calories. No more high fats and loads of simple sugars. No more addiction to fast, convenient junk foods. No more humongous portions. No more daily desserts and sweets. No more buckets of sweet carbonated beverages. No more binge drinking. That's the down side.

You also say, Yes to exercise! Yes to active participation! Yes to aerobics in some form or other! Yes to daily walking! You know you'll feel better. You know you'll look better. Best of all, you know you'll be healthier. So, that's the lifestyle you choose.

This way you set your first target. Maybe it's just that very first ten pounds. You go on your diet program and you go through your own *weight loss success cycle* and you achieve that ... so you celebrate! But then you go for your next ten pounds, and then the next, until you reach your target goal. Remember, to lose ten percent of your pre-diet weight is the first ideal target. When that is achieved, you may opt to target maintenance and govern your complete lifestyle accordingly. Or you may choose if you really had quite a bit to lose, to set a second target of another five or ten percent. Now, you're in a groove. You are exhilarated by results and you stay the course.

YOU WIN!

Now, you are ready to make your own personal application of **The Enzyme Diet™ Solution.** It really is quite easy.

☙

AS EASY AS 1-2-3

· **The Enzyme Diet™** is a delicious, healthy, low-fat meal replacement that uses the power of enzymes to reset your metabolism to its optimum level without drugs or stimulants.

• **The Enzyme Diet™** supplies your body with the essential enzymes, minerals, amino acids, carbohydrates, fatty acids, fiber, phytonutrients and natural vitamins needed to support your metabolism during weight loss.

• **The Enzyme Diet™** also provides a proprietary nutrient delivery system to ensure that these nutrients are absorbed and delivered to the cells with maximum efficiency. The result is safe and efficient weight loss, increased energy and overall improved health - with no drugs, stimulants or synthetic ingredients. Your personal Application is as easy as **1-2-3**:

☙ The Enzyme Diet™ Solution ☙

1. **To lose weight the healthy way:** Replace two meals a day, each with a delicious Enzyme Diet™ shake. Then eat a sensible and enjoyable third meal, one designed for completeness and balance.

2. **To maintain your lean muscle mass:** Exercise daily for 30 minutes or more, drink plenty of water (8 glasses per day) and enjoy fresh fruits or raw vegetables as snacks.

3. **To maintain your weight loss:** Then replace one meal a day with a delicious Enzyme Diet™ shake and eat sensibly the rest of the day. If you gain a few pounds, return to the weight loss plan (repeat actions 1 and 2) until you reach your desired weight.

If you want to lose weight and you are under 18, pregnant, nursing, following a diet recommended by a doctor, have health problems or want to lose more than 30 pounds, you should see a doctor before starting this or any other diet. Aim to lose no more than two pounds a week after the first week. Rapid weight loss may cause health problems. Do not use as a sole source of nutrition. Eat at least 1,200 calories a day.

Getting Started

In so many human endeavors, the hardest thing at times is to get started. You can think about what you want to do, talk about it, have all the good intentions to do it, but just put it off or even simply avoid it. Procrastinators tend to drift on a twin bed of indifference to their true status and an insensitivity to the demands of responsibility and opportunity before them. So although you really need to lose weight, you can deny any implications to your health or even your appearance and likewise profess that it's not your problem anyway. You can go through this steady sequence of denial, rationalization and default until you miss your chance and arrive at a point of resignation and regret. You can make excuses, continue to blame everything and everybody else and lose out on your life's best.

Are you a procrastinator? Have you been planning to do something about your weight for a long time, but you've really not changed anything? You think you have lots of time or it's just not that important. You have too many more important things to attend to. Perhaps you think your weight problem will just go away, or maybe you have got to the point where you don't care anymore.

So how will you get started? Here are some clues:

1. Choose a Specific Date. It makes sense to use a date that is significant to you. A birthday or anniversary is ideal but if that is too far away, choose one of your kids birthdays or your spouse's. How about a graduation date or immediately after a big event. Perhaps New Year's Day or a public holiday. The day the clocks change over in Spring or Fall. Maybe next Sunday, as it starts a new week. Or the first day of the next month. What specific date coming up might be significant for you? Then pin it down and make that choice.

2. Set an Initial Target. As we already pointed out, you want to aim to lose about ten percent of your pre-diet weight. But that's not the initial target. First you must take the little steps. To see your weight go down in the first week or two would be great. As long as it moves in the right direction, you've made a start. Then put a benchmark at your first five or ten pounds off. Then go for five or ten more, and perhaps five or ten more. Those little steps all add up. You will approach your real target.

3. Clean out your Refrigerator/Freezer. You will eat whatever you buy and take home. Your refrigerator and freezer are full of what you and your family plan to eat. So it's no use going on a specific low calorie weight loss program, only to open your refrigerator or freezer every day to look at all those dense calories and high fat foods. Frozen desserts galore are irresistible. Lead yourself not into temptation. Remove the temptations. Eat them first before you decide to lose weight or better still, give them away. It's a new day, a new beginning - you're in search of a New YOU.

4. Go to a new Supermarket. We're all creatures of habit. If you've shopped at the same supermarket for any length of time, you now have routines. You know where everything is, at least all the items you usually buy. You follow common aisles in some kind of sequence and you see only what you want to see. You tend to buy the same things almost every time. A typical supermarket has close to 10,000 different items on its shelves, but the typical family purchases only about 200 or 300 food items repeatedly. No more. That's your supermarket within the supermarket. That has to change if you want to lose weight. So find a new place to buy the new goods you now choose to focus on to become the New YOU. Specialize on new items in new aisles. Do not shop when you are hungry but when you are full. Begin now, always in the vegetable and fruit aisles. Avoid the junk food and soda pop aisles. Read the labels. Reduce your food budget by ten or twenty percent. Take a notebook with you to this new place and make notes of everything you buy. You'll review this later and make further changes. But remember, you will always eat what you buy, so be careful about what you buy.

5. Buy a new pair of Sneakers. You may need another pair of sneakers as much as you need more clothes to add to those that already can't fit you, or can't fit in your overcrowded cupboards. You have shoes and sandals of every description. So why a new pair of sneakers? Did you know that Michael Jordan made a habit of wearing new basketball shoes for every game. Why? He told Oprah he wanted to make each game special. You want to make your weight loss program special and you want to make exercise a special part of that program. One certain way to do that is to get new sneakers. They will encourage you to go walking, perhaps jogging or even back to the gym. But they should get you off the couch.

6. Rearrange your TV room. Speaking of getting off the couch, you want to change your entertainment routines too. Television is an enemy of many things, including effective weight loss. You have TV habits: your favorite programs, your favorite shows, your favorite place to recline and even your favorite snacks and drinks for when you put your feet up. That's not consistent with what you're trying to do. So it makes sense to change. Therefore, rearrange your furniture, evaluate which TV programs to drop first, and choose new snacks of raw vegetables and fruit, etc.

7. Buy a Weigh Scale. Here's something real practical. You want to be weight conscious and you want to monitor your progress. You don't have to be extravagant, for your success is not affected by the scale. It's vice versa. If you don't have a working scale, get an economical one from your local store and keep it in view in your bathroom. But a word of caution: don't become paranoid. No weight measurement on any given day really means anything. It's only the trend down over periods of time that matters. Expect some minor daily variations. That's just noise. Stick to your program and you'll see results.

8. Date the Notches on your Belt. Another practical idea. Inside your belt, put a date to mark the hole you now use to buckle up. As you lose weight, your waist will go down - first an inch, then two, then three and so on, depending on where you get started. That could be exciting for you.

9. Purchase The Enzyme Diet™. That's easy. Talk to the person who orginally told you about **The Enzyme Diet™** book or product. You can also order directly on the Internet at www.infinity2.com and click on the country you live in to order this product. This is the e-commerce generation, after all. As you apply your **Enzyme Diet™ Solution** you will use this as a substitute for breakfast and lunch each day. You'll especially need four canisters per month - a good starter order.

10. Post your Daily Routine. You must devise a plan for a typical day as you apply your **Enzyme Diet™ Solution**. **Table 7** is a suggested outline that allows you to enjoy healthful, low calorie snacks between meals and a sensible dinner. A variety of dinner recipes will be described in the next chapter. Similarly, an exercise routine will be described in Ch 9.

Table 7.   A typical day for **The Enzyme Diet™ Solution**

Breakfast	1 Enzyme Diet Shake
Optional Snack	1 medium size fruit such as an apple, pear or orange
Lunch	1 Enzyme Diet Shake
Optional Snack	1 cup fresh vegetables with low fat dip or 1 cup nonfat yogurt or 1 cup low fat soup
Dinner	4 to 6 oz poultry, fish or lean meat (cooked weight) or vegetarian equivalent, 1/2 baked potato or 1/2 cup whole grain pasta or brown rice 3 vegetables, large salad (See Chapter 8 - Recipes)
Optional Snack	1/2 cup berries with 1 cup nonfat yogurt

Exercise Routine: e.g. Choose one or more of the following to suit your exercise level:
* Walk 30 minutes after dinner
* Swim Wednesday evenings and Saturday mornings
* Aerobics Monday, Wednesday and Friday
* Super Slow workout Tuesday, Thursday and Saturday (See Chapter 9 - Exercise)

Keep it simple. Stick to your plan. Be accountable and have fun! It really is:

As Easy as 1-2-3!

and

As Simple as A-B-C!

AS SIMPLE AS   A - B - C

Losing weight is not rocket science. It's a simple lifestyle habit that yields results. It comes down to some pretty basic things. Yes, it's as simple as A-B-C:

A ttitude

+

B ehavior

+

C onsistency

A.   Your ATTITUDE is paramount. Begin by accepting yourself. Affirm yourself as a person - not a body, not a weight. Just a person. Fat is not a personality trait. It's something you carry just now, but it's not you. It's certainly not the important thing about you. And that you're going to lose. You'll look better perhaps and you'll feel better too, but you'll be no better just because you've lost some extra weight. The essence of you won't really change. Therefore, your present self-image can be just as positive and strong now as you hope it will be after you've lost your weight. Keep that positive attitude throughout. Believe you can because you really can!

B.   Your BEHAVIOR will determine your results. Weight loss that is effective and persistent is always the result of permanent lifestyle modification. Good eating habits, moderate but increased physical activity and the judicious use of **The Enzyme Diet**™ to replace breakfast and lunch is the way to go. Action produces results. Make your actions deliberate and avoid impulsive eating. Remain physically active and resist the inertia of lethargy. You will see on the scales the sum total of all your daily lifestyle choices. Therefore you need to practice doing the right thing!

C.   Your CONSISTENCY is the key. Think about this. It is not what you do very occasionally that defines your lifestyle or the quality of your life. Rather, it's what you do each and every day. Therefore, every time you mix **The Enzyme Diet**™ in your shaker or blender for breakfast or lunch, you're losing weight. Every time you choose a snack of fresh fruit or raw vegetables instead of potato chips or soda pop, you're losing weight. Every time you sit down for your sensible dinner that's got variety but relatively low fat or calories, you're losing weight. Every time you go for a long walk or swim two laps in the pool, or exercise in the gym, you're losing weight. It is the sum total of those consistent choices that will give you results. **A-B-C.** That's how you attain your goal!

ATTITUDE + BEHAVIOR + CONSISTENCY = RESULTS

Tips For Maximizing Your Results

1.   Create sensible dinner meals
A sensible meal is low in fat and sugar, includes plenty of raw vegetables and fiber, and has a moderate amount of carbohydrates and protein. Your meal choices can be varied. However, including a combination of the following foods and suggested serving sizes may greatly enhance your weight loss efforts.

As a guide, feel free to choose foods that fit these general requirements:

- 4-6 ounces of lean meat (chicken, turkey, white meat fish - including tuna in water) or ½ - 1 c. beans, soy protein, cottage cheese, miso or tofu
- 1-2 tbsp raw fat (avocado, raw nuts and seeds)
- 1-2 servings of whole grains (serving = 1 slice bread, ½ roll, 1/3 c. rice or ½ c. pasta)
- 2-4 servings of vegetables (1c. raw {preferably} or ½ c. cooked)
A number of original recipes will be given in the next chapter.

2.   Choose some healthy snacks
If you find yourself feeling hungry between meals, the very best snack you can have is another serving of **The Enzyme Diet**™. Some people,

however, feel more satisfied if they chew something. If this is the case with you, we recommend raw fruits and vegetables. Make these readily available. To optimize weight loss, you will want to limit your snacks to two per day.

3.   Create a realistic vision of how you want to look and feel
The mind has an amazing capacity to direct the body. You become what you think about all day, and you can direct your thoughts so you can accomplish the things you desire most. By creating a clear vision of how you want to look and feel, you will find it easier to achieve your weight loss goals. As Walt Disney said: *'Imagination is the preview of all life's coming attractions.'*

4.   Drink eight glasses of water each day
Drinking plenty of water daily promotes healthy functioning of all the body's systems and encourages further weight loss. Being dehydrated can sabotage your weight loss efforts and your metabolism. Many Americans mistake thirst for hunger, which can cause dieters to overeat. If you think you're hungry between your allotted meals and snacks, drink a glass of water. An easy way to track your water intake is to fill up 2 or 3 one-liter bottles of water each day and be sure to drink them before the end of the day. Juices and other sweetened beverages add significant amounts of calories and sugar to your diet. In fact, 12 ounces of juice has more calories than a serving of **The Enzyme Diet™**. If you do drink juice, make sure to count it toward one of your daily snacks and be sure it is freshly squeezed.

5.   Avoid all carbonated beverages
Carbonated beverages are typically high in sugar and their consumption is linked to increased obesity and diabetes rates in the United States. Even if the beverage contains no sugar, the carbonation destroys enzymes and the friendly intestinal bacteria required for healthy digestion and immunity. The carbonation destroys the active enzymes contained in **The Enzyme Diet™** too. Without these enzymes, **The Enzyme Diet™** cannot properly support your metabolism and promote weight loss. So, even though diet soda has no calories, it can sabotage your weight loss efforts and affect your health.

6.   Refrain from eating 2-3 hours before bedtime
Your metabolism drops significantly at night, causing the body to store calories as fat rather than use them as energy. Also, many people tend to do the most snacking while relaxing in front of the TV at night. Breaking this habit will be a positive lifestyle change long after you have achieved your weight loss goals.

7.   Increase your physical activity
Doing any type of aerobic activity (walking, cycling, running, swimming, aerobic dance, stair climbing, in-line skating, etc.) for about 30 minutes three times a week is ideal and will greatly enhance your weight loss efforts. You should also add strength training to your routine three times a week (on the alternate days) to help you replace fat with muscle and further enhance your metabolism. If you are not used to exercising, begin slowly with a 20-minute walk to build up your endurance. As the pounds come off, you will find exercising easier to do.

8.   Use nutritional supplements daily
The Enzyme Diet™ was designed for a specific purpose - to keep your metabolism high, while consuming a low number of calories. By adding other nutritional supplements, you can allow your body to help digest and absorb the healthy meals and snacks you consume in addition to **The Enzyme Diet™**. The more nutrients you take in, the more energy (stored fat/calories) your body will be able to burn.

9.   Treat yourself occasionally
You deserve a break - not every day, but occasionally you must allow yourself the pure delight of enjoying something you really love to eat even if it does not quite belong in your **Enzyme Diet™** Daily Routine Plan. Make a list of four or five things that you know will really appeal to you because you enjoy them so much. Schedule occasional indulgence rather than do it on impulse when you have an emotional need. You do it when you choose to and not when you need to. That way you maintain discipline and control. You're not being punished or deprived, especially if you have intentions for long term maintenance. The art of discipline here is moderation and balance. Give yourself permission and enjoy the treat while it lasts. Then go back immediately to your structured routine without any sense of guilt. You will still achieve your goal.

10.   Control your impulses as your mood changes
You must find alternative ways of coping with your feelings. Go for a walk, play an instrument, have a warm bath, do some shopping, write a poem, go visit a friend ... do something else - anything but eat. This will bring deliverance from any subtle addictions to food that you may have and any tendency to that form of escapism. That is true behavior modification which must take place for any long term success at weight loss.

Your Exit Strategy

The way you exit your diet is critical to your long-term success. Millions of people begin weight loss programs each year. Many of them are successful in achieving their desired weight, but few are successful at *maintaining* that weight loss over the long term. The key reasons why so many find it so hard to maintain the early weight loss are:

i.   The type of diet they used to obtain the results;

ii.   The way they "exit" the diet, and

iii. The failure to plan.

Although these sound like different issues, they are actually one issue - healthy habits. Naturally, the failure to plan is a plan to fail. Therefore, the diet must be carefully selected and the necessary exit strategy skillfully executed. If the diet used to achieve weight loss failed to develop healthy habits, the individual will be unlikely to maintain the diet. Examples of diets that do not develop healthy habits include: diets that promote eliminating entire food groups; diets that promote eating only one food (even if the food is nutritious) such as grapefruit or cabbage soup; using stimulants, fat blockers or fat substitutes; and diets that are nothing more than just diets.

Not only do these diets fail to help you develop healthy habits, but they also ruin metabolic rate. Diets that limit food groups, simply cut calories or rely on fake nutrients, fat blockers or stimulants do not supply the body with the nutrients needed to maintain metabolism. The result is a reduced metabolic rate that causes you to gain the weight back even when you continue to eat very small amounts.

Similarly, if you fail to maintain healthy habits established during the weight loss period or "diet" period, then you will also be unlikely to maintain the weight loss. Returning to unhealthy eating habits also sabotages metabolism and makes it difficult to maintain the weight loss.

The key healthy lifestyle habits that should be part of your weight loss strategy and should be included as part of your exit strategy should include the following:

1. **Eat 5 servings of fresh fruits and vegetables each day.**

2. **Drink at least eight glasses of water each day.**

3. **Do at least 20 minutes of moderate physical activity daily.**

4. **Eat four to six small meals and snacks throughout the day rather than two or three large meals.**

5. **Eat whole grains such as whole wheat, bran, oat and rye breads, pastas and cereals and brown rice.**

6. **Limit intake of saturated fat (e.g. fried foods, red meats and dairy), alcohol, caffeine and carbonated beverages.**

7. **Limit your intake of sweets/desserts to once a week.**

8. **Maintain an active interest in weight and wellness.**

9. **Remain accountable to yourself and others.**

10. **Monitor your weight regularly (chart).**

Following these simple habits will make it easier to obtain and maintain a healthy weight. They will also keep your body healthy, with more energy and vitality to enjoy life.

ૐ   YOUR EXIT STRATEGY   ૐ

What you do as you transition from weight loss to weight management is what is frequently referred to as 'the exit strategy'. This strategy is key to maintaining the weight loss you worked so hard to achieve.

Your Exit Strategy continues to be **As Simple as 1-2-3**:

1.
Monitor Your Weight Regularly:
If you notice a two or three pounds creeping up on the scale, then simply resume your previous weight loss plan (assuming you chose a healthy weight loss plan like **The Enzyme Diet™ Solution** that maintains metabolism). Losing two or three pounds is much easier than losing twenty or thirty. That's common sense at work.

2.
Continue the Healthy Habits:
These include both the Diet and the Exercise Routines you developed while achieving your weight loss goals. Deliberate choices initiate actions; consistent actions become habits; combined habits define a lifestyle; and a healthy lifestyle will yield the NEW YOU.

3.
Keep it Off for Life:
Simply replace one meal a day with a delicious shake of **The Enzyme Diet™** and eat sensibly the rest of the day. This lifestyle will ensure that your metabolism continues to run at optimum rate. If you gain a few pounds, return to the weight loss plan until you reach your desired weight.

The Enzyme Diet™ Solution is not just a diet, but a lifetime of health. It is designed to optimize metabolism and ensure that you not only obtain your goals, but also maintain them. Unlike typical low-calorie diets where your metabolism drops as much as 30% in the first two weeks, **The Enzyme Diet™** optimizes your metabolism and ensures that your metabolism is functioning at a more optimum level than when you began.

Because you don't sacrifice your metabolism while you're on **The Enzyme Diet™** , you won't feel that you need to "eat everything in sight" when you reach your goal weight. You'll have the energy you need to enjoy life and you won't experience the bounce back weight gain because you haven't deprived your body of the essential nutrition it needs and your metabolism isn't sluggish.

It's a world of difference compared to "typical" low calorie diets. **The Enzyme Diet™ Solution** is designed with an appropriate exit strategy for lasting results. The meal replacement shake can be used daily for a lifetime to provide all the nutrients the body needs to optimize metabolism - complex carbohydrates, protein, essential fats, enzymes, whole food vitamins, minerals and other phytonutrients.

With this exit strategy - you drink one shake a day to keep your metabolism functioning at the optimum level. You'll want to make **The Enzyme Diet™** a part of your daily life because of the way you feel. When you feel better, healthier and more energetic after losing weight, it's easy to make better choices for yourself. But when you complete a diet that is unhealthy and lacking nutrition you feel tired and cranky. With 'brain fog' and fatigue associated with a lack of nutrition, you're more inclined to reach for comfort food to help with the diet blues than to go for a walk or make healthy food choices.

Losing weight with **The Enzyme Diet™ Solution** isn't torture like other diets. With this program you will supply your body with more nutrition than it normally gets and, in return, your body will respond by giving you more energy, better sleep, healthier skin, a clear mind and a better outlook. Instead of looking in the mirror and seeing a drawn, gaunt face (which often happens when losing weight with so many other diets) - you'll not only be thinner but you'll look and feel younger and healthier.

Well, guess what? It's time to **Design your own Menu**.

❧ *Chapter 8* ❧

DESIGN YOUR OWN MENU
Eat Right. Feel Right

    You need to design your own weight loss menu. Therefore, in this chapter, you will receive the tools to easily implement a program of good nutrition to complement **The Enzyme Diet™**. You will understand the basics of good nutrition, learn how to set up your kitchen to promote health, and receive the menus, recipes and shopping guidelines to quickly get started. You will also find suggestions for eating at your favorite fast-food establishments and restaurants without increasing your weight or compromising your health.

    You already know that *what you eat* is a most crucial consideration. More importantly, you should always focus on *what your cells eat*. That's the result you recall, of the Seven Steps of nutrition, including the obvious ingestion and digestion as the first two steps. The principles of proper ingestion and digestion will be at the root of most recommendations we will make in this chapter. The foods to choose and the preparation methods to be described are those that promote healthy digestion and nutrient delivery.

    At the outset, we recommend that you observe the so-called *Ten Commandments of Good Nutrition*. These basics discussed below should become 'laws' in your own personal commitment to general health and to effective weight loss in particular. Use these recommendations as a beginning, then stick to them faithfully. They arrest some of the biggest culprits when it comes to the influence of nutrition on disease and ill health. Don't let your own lack of will power, your busy schedule, your vacations or anything else get in the way of this giant step toward better health and your own personal victory in managing your weight satisfactorily. Following these simple suggestions will free you from many health hazards.

❦

TEN COMMANDMENTS OF GOOD NUTRITION

Commandment #1. Eat Small, Regular and Varied Meals

Unlike some other animals, humans have relatively small stomachs designed for small, frequent meals.

Small means exactly what it says: small. Americans eat too much. The portions served in restaurants and fast food places in particular have become embarrassingly huge. Competition and cheap food technology have given the consumer the windfall benefit of overflowing 14 and 16 inch plates, 16 oz and 20 oz steaks and 20 and 24 oz tumblers of sweet sodas and pop to wash the largesse down. The bad habits have been taken home and domestic kitchens now prepare the same huge barbecue steaks and burgers, overflowing bowls of soup and stew and heaps of rice and mashed potatoes. Whatever became of fine dining with its respectful, delicately placed apologies for each portion of every course? Whatever became of meals centered around vegetables, salads and fruits?

Typically, **The Enzyme Diet™ Solution** calls for light regular dinners of just 4 to 6 ounces for cooked portions of poultry, fish or lean meat, or some vegetarian equivalent. Add this to half a baked potato or half a cup of whole grain pasta or brown rice for example, combined with 3 vegetables in any style, and a large salad. **The Enzyme Diet™** meal replacement shake adequately serves for breakfast and lunch, while light snacks of fresh fruit or any vegetables round off the daily fare.

Regular eating has gone the way of the dinosaur. But if you are to lose weight effectively and regain control of your health status, you must adopt a new lifestyle pattern to include fairly regular meals.

Varied implies balancing the menu from all sections of the Eating Right Pyramid (**Fig. 2**). It is a visual representation of how to eat foods in a healthy ratio. By following the Food Pyramid, your food intake each day should be about 60 percent carbohydrates, 20 percent protein and 20 percent fat. Everyone should eat this way. These same ratios are recommended for old and young alike. At the end of the day, you should be able to look at what you have eaten and see that it generally fits this Food Pyramid principle.

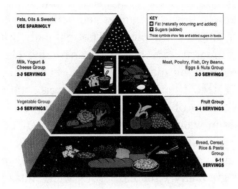

Fig 2.   The Eating Right Food Pyramid (USDA)

Commandment #2. Drink at least Eight Glasses of Fluid Each Day

Adequate fluid intake is a necessary healthy habit, especially during a weight loss program.   On a daily basis, a normal healthy adult loses about 2.6 litres (approximately 85 ounces, 10 cups) of fluid loss each day.   This needs to be replaced by at least eight glasses of fluid of one kind or another.

When it comes to fluid intake, Americans also get it wrong. We drink all the wrong fluids in abundance: carbonated beverages, coffee or tea, and alcoholic drinks. We seek to quench our thirst in all the unhealthy places. Carbonated beverages you learned in the last chapter are high in refined sugar which means empty calories. Even the diet versions without sugar tend to destroy the active enzymes present in **The Enzyme Diet**™ and in the secreted juices of the stomach and intestine. That's in part, why even people who drink "diet" sodas still seem to have trouble losing weight.

Coffee and tea are usually caffeinated and that has all the associated detrimental consequences. Alcohol hardly necessitates comment. Although there is good reported evidence for some positive health benefits attributed to red wine in moderation, the net effects of alcohol in the body, in the home and in society are large and unequivocally negative.

Therefore, it is both wise and convenient for the population at large, but for dieters in particular, to choose much healthier alternatives for fluid consumption. What are your options? **Water is probably best,**

and you need plenty of it. Find a good source and make that a common daily habit. In addition, fresh fruit juices and perhaps some skim milk (if you can tolerate it) should complete your normal daily drink routine.

With an estimated 75% of Americans being chronically dehydrated, chances are drinking more water could help you in your weight loss efforts. You'll need even more if you exercise more. You should drink an extra 4-6 ounces of water for every 15 minutes of exercise, and an extra two glasses of water for every glass of alcohol, coffee or tea that you indulge in, if you insist.

If you are not used to drinking this much water, you may want to make this change gradually. Increase your water intake by one eight ounce glass each day until you reach the recommended amounts.

Commandment #3. Favor Foods With Low Glycemic Index
(Cutback on Refined Sugars)

The Glycemic Index concept was mentioned in Chapter 2. It measures the speed at which you digest food and convert it into glucose, the essential energy fuel of your body. The faster the food breaks down, the higher the rating on the index. The index or scale sets simple sugar itself (pure glucose) at 100 and scores all foods against that number. Professor David Jenkins first published an index in 1980, showing the various rates at which different carbohydrate foods break down and release glucose into the blood stream. New standard international tables were published in the *American Journal of Clinical Nutrition* in 1995 [1].

Low glycemic foods promote a slow, moderate rise in blood sugars and insulin levels after a meal. This helps keep hunger in check and encourages the body to dissolve body fat by converting it to energy. In contrast, high glycemic foods cause sudden, unstable swings in blood sugar. The end result is an increase in appetite and irritability, and a greater tendency to convert food calories into body fat.

As a standard routine of **The Enzyme Diet™ Solution**, you are encouraged to include a lot of low and medium glycemic foods in your diet. Also, whenever you eat a high glycemic food, combine it with a food from the low glycemic list in order to help balance the effects. Following this aspect of the plan will help minimize hunger and will reduce the tendency to overeat, thus helping you lose body fat. Even for those whose main objective is not fat loss, low glycemic foods will help alleviate mood swings and regulate energy levels. A recent study has shown the benefits of a low glycemic index diet for diabetes and for weight loss.

Commandment #4. Run Away From Fat

The Enzyme Diet™ Solution recommends that you watch the percentage of fat in your foods. No more than 20 percent of your total caloric intake should be from fat. That implies avoiding fat wherever it is clearly visible in your diet. Use only lean cuts of meat. Remove the fatty skins from poultry and fish. Skim all the fats and oils from the surface of cooked foods, canned preparations, refrigerated and frozen foods whenever visible. Eliminate fried foods. Although fat is necessary in your diet, the fat in fried foods is enzyme deficient, so it cannot be readily used for energy in your body. Therefore, instead of eating fried foods, you can steam, bake or broil your foods. Better yet, eat them raw when possible. Avoid bacon and sausage. Go light on butter and use only skimmed dairy products. When you purchase packaged foods, read the labels and select low fat items carefully.

Most consumers are now aware that high fat consumption is generally unhealthy. There has been a distinct trend to reduce fat consumption but food manufacturers and marketers are not to be outdone. Therefore, they have created a new industry of low fat foods. Unfortunately, you can't rely on the advertised percentages to paint a true picture for you. Labels that boast "98 percent fat free" or "50 percent less fat" are misleading. The fat percentages on these labels are based on volume only. For example, if you were to take a bottle of water and put one drop of oil in it, you could say that by volume, the water is 99 percent fat free. Yet, based on calories, it is 100 percent fat.

What about foods without labels? Many foods, such as raw fruits and vegetables, fish and poultry do not have labels. These are all less than 20% fat. On the other hand, beef, whole dairy, pork, fats and oils are at 60% fat or more.

Even though it is prudent to reduce dietary fat, one must always remember the need for essential fatty acids as pointed out in chapter 6. In addition, all fats are not equal. Aim to avoid trans-fatty acids and the more harmful hydrogenated fats and oils, whenever you have a choice.

Commandment #5. Eat as many Raw Foods As Possible

Foods in their natural raw state contain many nutrients that have been identified. However, there are certain unknown components in raw foods that make them more beneficial than foods that are cooked, processed, or altered from their natural state in any way. Along with these unknown healthy components that are lost, there are vital nutrients that we do know about that are destroyed when foods are cooked or processed. They include enzymes.

According to nature's plan, enzymes that occur naturally in foods are supposed to help digest that food and break it down in the body. When we eat cooked or processed foods, the only way that those foods can be digested is to draw on digestive enzymes from the body's supply. We referred to this problem back in Chapter 4. The body's ability to produce digestive enzymes is limited and can become depleted. Like an enzyme bank account, we make withdrawals from our enzyme supply when we eat foods that are cooked or processed.

When our supply of digestive enzymes is exhausted, to accomplish the process of digestion, the body then robs from its reserve of metabolic enzymes that are supposed to be used for other functions.

In addition to the loss of digestive enzymes and valuable nutrients, another consideration when focused on the necessity for raw foods, is the great importance of fiber. Raw foods especially green leafy vegetables, fruits, cereals and grains, all tend to be rich in fiber. Soluble fibers have been shown to be important in glucose tolerance, particularly the complex carbohydrate foods with their low glycemic index. These same fibers prove effective in binding cholesterol in the gut and help reduce serum cholesterol - a significant factor in cardiovascular disease.

Fiber also provides the necessary indigestible bulk to the diet to favor bowel health in a wide variety of ways.

Therefore, **The Enzyme Diet™ Solution** recommends that you stick with grains that come directly from the earth. Select whole grains and pasta which are higher in fiber than the processed white flour products which are depleted, bleached and refined for commercial advantages and profits. Eat raw fruits and fresh vegetables also for their fiber content. After all, high fiber foods are more satisfying.

Since you can't always eat raw foods, take a plant based digestive enzyme supplement, and use a whole food vitamin/chelated mineral supplement to ensure your adequate nutrition.

Commandment #6. Shop For Health

Imagine that every time you went into your local supermarket or wherever you shop for food, you saw a sign over the main entrance that read:

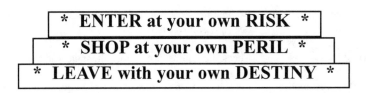

Or how about a flashing amber light outside the front door, with a large posted neon sign that said -

CAUTION: You will Become What You Buy Here!

That might as well be posted there. Both warnings are true. You eat whatever you buy and you become whatever your cells eat. Therefore , you should always be careful what foods you buy. It is disturbing to realize that the body you have today was reconstructed only from the foods you bought and consumed over the past few years. The same will be true looking forward, so the struggle for good health and certainly controlled weight will continue to be fought in the aisles of your super-market.

Shop at your leisure, only when you're in a good mood and have time to discriminate. Leave the kids at home, if possible. Their influence could be deadly. Avoid shopping when you're hungry and more gullible to sensual appeals to your appetite. Begin always at the vegetable and fruit aisles. Move systematically through the market if possible and avoid some aisles altogether - those with junk food and highly processed, convenience foods. Focus on the nutritional content of foods, with a goal to maximize the essential nutrients. Reduce the calories, simple sugars and fat, and also increase the fiber. Specialize in all foods that can be eaten raw, in their naturally occurring state. As we pointed out before, raw foods supply essential vitamins and minerals and contain the enzymes necessary to aid in the digestion of those foods. In fact, a suggested order of preference for your food selections is given in **Table 8**.

Table 8.   Order of Preference For Food Selections

1. **Raw.** — This is the best and most nutritious offering. Rich in enzymes.

2. **Frozen or Dried.** — Without preservatives and at low temperatures. Freezing does not destroy enzymes.

3. **Bottled Raw.** — Check the liquids, if any, for salt, sugar and preservatives.

4. **Lightly Sweetened.** — Look for hidden sources of sugar. Avoid sugar substitutes.

5. **Baked.** — Choose low fat wherever possible.

6. **Reduced** — For quick sale. Usually natural foods, but not fresh. Often stale dated. Decreased nutritional value.

7. **Canned.** — Not the most preferred healthy alternative.

8. **Preserved.** — Loaded with chemicals and additives for extended shelf life.

9. **Microwaved.** — Never recommended.

10. **Synthetic.** — Some food items are not foods at all. Avoid.

Commandment #7. Avoid Crash Diets

Crash diets will make you crash! It's that simple. It's that unhealthy.

We referred earlier to the most guaranteed weight loss diet - put duct tape to cover the mouth and keep it there. With that method, you must lose weight. That's for sure. But you will also lose your health and if you were to persist, you would die.

Crash diets are only a variation of that approach. Very low calorie diets that make no provision for the essential nutritional needs of the body cannot be adhered to for long before serious consequences follow. The history of this industry has been given several black marks at times when different promoters have unwisely but successfully captured the interest of frustrated, ill-informed dieters. In their desperation, many resorted to one of these crash diets only to eventually crash. They often saw early dramatic results as their bodies moved into a true 'starvation' mode. They lost water quickly and then began to burn both their lean muscle mass and their unwanted fat. But as their cells starved, their metabolism slowed, their biochemistry became toxic, their liver and kidneys began to fail, their energy declined and before you knew it, they became very ill and, in some unfortunate cases, they were victims of premature death. What a ghastly scenario to contemplate.

In extreme cases, where rapid weight loss may be indicated, it should always be done under medical supervision. You should be very suspicious and in fact, avoid following any diet independently that offers less than 1,000 to 1,200 calories per day. You'd be destined to crash, sooner or later.

Crash diets starve the body of unwanted calories but also of essential nutrients. Crash diets are unnatural and unsatisfying. They cannot be maintained indefinitely. Crash diets are manipulative, almost passive-aggressive choices. They avoid underlying personal and social issues. Crash diets necessitate no fundamental changes. They are therefore self defeating. Crash diets are unhealthy. They always fail!

Commandment #8. Practice only responsible fasting

Fasting is the voluntary abstinence from solid food over any period of time out of the ordinary. *It is not dieting* and should not be related to dieting per se! Just the thought of decreased quantity of food - not to mention *no food* - over any unusual period of time, is enough to strike terror into the hearts of many people. Those addicted to their food (and in large quantities) must consider any suggestion of fasting to be off their radar screens. But not so fast, it does make sense when practiced correctly and it does have its place in modern culture. Fasting has often been abused by dieters and it is not a requirement of **The Enzyme Diet™ Solution** program per se, but this optional habit has its place when used responsibly.

If you think about it, our normal daily eating routine begins with a break-fast. That is correct terminology because under normal circumstances, we undergo a brief, limited fast overnight. We effectively rest our stomachs and intestines and give them a chance to recuperate from all the demands we impose during the day, with the wide variety of foods we ingest under a variety of stressful circumstances. In that sense, we fast each night and break the fast with the addition of food in the morning.

That same principle which seems so natural, could be occasionally exploited for your own benefit. The suggested idea would be to incorporate into your dietary program, an occasional - perhaps monthly - interruption of your normal dietary habits. You have a regular, light dinner or supper and then have no solid foods, but drink copious amounts of only clear fluids (water itself is best), for the next 18 to 24 hours. During that time, the fluids purge the gut and aid the liver and kidneys to eliminate waste metabolites and any soluble pollutants that you may have accumulated in your system.

At the end of this short liquid fast, you reintroduce other foods, first with a serving of **The Enzyme Diet**™ or even a light snack, and then a few hours later, you may resume your normal diet with a light balanced meal.

This idea of a regular fast on fluids only is not recommended for small children, diabetics or those clinically ill or under medical management. But it is a healthy recommendation particularly for those who are on the maintenance phase of a sensible weight loss dietary program, particularly **The Enzyme Diet**™ **Solution.**

Commandment #9. Occasionally Treat Yourself

Eating is a necessity but it should also be a pleasure. A healthy diet must invariably be a fun diet, or else it is not a true diet, but rather a self-inflicted punishment. Whatever limitations you arrive at - whether restricting calories, reducing fat, avoiding junk food, eating at home exclusively, eliminating certain foods, eating lesser quantities, substituting meals, taking short fasts, or whatever else - you must make room for eating *with* pleasure and *for* pleasure. Food is something to be enjoyed.

So many people start out on a new diet, enjoying the results. They're looking good and feeling good. But it only lasts a couple months and then, it's back to the unhealthy eating as usual. They cannot be so 'masochistic' forever. At coffee break, first they itch for some sweet delight that others seem to enjoy, but they would have none of it. Initial discipline to resist is a source of pride and offers protection from the unthinkable, sinful capitulation. Then they become tense and irritable; later stoic and angry; finally desperate, resigned and eventually indulgent. More often than not, they become recklessly so, and indifferent to the consequences. Such people are invariably too hard on themselves - before, during and after the entire futile exercise.

You must choose a different course. Cultivate dietary habits that are rational, reasonable and rewarding in terms of both pleasure and weight management.

What are your favorite foods? Do you have a favorite place to eat? Have you marked special items in the supermarket as yours to enjoy? It would make good sense for you to determine in advance what those are, and then to allow yourself a quota. You may choose to include your treats as a regular part of your weekly menu. Or you may choose to use your treats as simple tokens of reward and recognition for your performance of physical activities that you identify, or the attainment of specific weight goals. In any case, do give yourself permission and avoid any guilt complex. If you over indulge at any time, correct your wayward indulgence with a new sacrifice that compensates. You can then either avoid a normal calorie item that would otherwise be included or else, constrain yourself to some additional quantum of exercise to burn those extra calories off. The bottom line is balance and discipline. Both extremes of deprivation and indulgence are bad, impractical and unhealthy in the long run. So govern yourself accordingly.

Commandment #10. Supplement Your Diet

Clinical nutrition is a specialized practice in the care and management of patients with diagnosed illness. Supplementation however, is a wise lifestyle alternative even for healthy individuals, to provide a guaranteed supply of *essential* nutrients to the body, on a regular basis, and in a convenient form. It is in essence, first and foremost, a form of *nutritional insurance*. We live in an age of busy lifestyles, an industrialized food supply, commonly poor food choices, and excessive demands from the stress and pollutants in our environment. It has become very difficult in contemporary society to find the ingredients for a truly healthy diet and to make consumption of the same a regular lifestyle pattern. Under such circumstances, you can make certain that you get what your cells need by the careful and responsible use of food supplements that provide all the basic essentials.

There are at least **Five Areas for Responsible Supplementation** that need to be addressed. These essentials are (i) Enzymes, (ii) Vitamins, (iii) Minerals, (iv) Antioxidants, and (v) Probiotics.

(i) **Enzymes**. As we saw in Chapter 4, digestive enzymes are found naturally in foods. They are present to initiate the process of digestion in the early fundus of the stomach. But they are destroyed by processing and cooking above 118 degrees F. That means the body must handle the extremely energy-consuming task of digestion by using its own limited enzyme supply. When the body is forced to handle the increased demands of digestion, its own enzymes can become depleted and chronic digestive problems and other health conditions increase.

Enzymes must therefore be replenished for proper digestion. They must also keep every other bodily process functioning optimally. Without adequate enzymes the body is overtaxed, we fatigue more easily, have more digestive problems, we are sick more often and we age more rapidly. Yet, supplementing with enzymes is easy. All you need to do is to take a good pure plant enzyme formula each time you eat cooked or processed food.

(ii) **Vitamins**. Essential vitamins are indispensable for life and health and must be consumed in one form or another. There are water soluble vitamins like vitamin C and B-complex (8 essentials), and fat soluble vitamins like vitamins A, D, E and K. These are all relatively small molecules present in minute amounts in the body, but they are critical for a wide variety of cellular functions. Among other things, they are important co-factors in many enzyme functions. Vitamin deficiency diseases like scurvy or pellagra are but extreme examples of how the body fails to function without adequate supply of vitamins.

Due to modern processing and growing methods, much of our current food supply is devoid of essential nutrients. Dietary choices and lifestyles show a distinct shift from all-natural whole foods to processed and convenience foods with far less vitamin content. Supplementation with whole food vitamins is a wise lifestyle choice to guarantee the essentials that your cells need every day. The CAeDS® nutrient delivery system would be an important ingredient in any high quality multi-vitamin supplement.

Natural source vitamins are superior to the synthetic isolates prepared synthetically in the laboratory. The natural vitamins occur in unique forms and structures that are difficult to reproduce. More importantly, they contain many more trace ingredients that complete a vitamin complex which optimizes their total nutritional value.

(iii) **Minerals**. The body needs a consistent supply of major and minor (trace) minerals for growth and metabolism. Much emphasis has been placed on calcium particularly for postmenopausal women who are prone to reduced bone density and pathological fractures as estrogen levels fall off. Similarly, where blood loss is significant, especially in women of child bearing age, iron deficiency anemia is not uncommon and supplementation becomes necessary. The need for trace minerals like zinc, chromium, magnesium, manganese, copper, cobalt, etc. is emphasized because studies have revealed an alarming decline in the mineral content of commercially grown foods. The refining process used to make breads, cereals and other grain products removes as much as 75% of the minerals and only a few are added back in the attempted fortification process.

Fruits and vegetables are convenient sources of both vitamins and minerals but only 9% of the American population consumes the recommended five servings of fruits and vegetables each day. The intake of milk and dairy products as a good source of calcium poses problems of lactose intolerance for some while others have questioned the health implications of both homogenization and pasteurization. Meats are a good source of iron but the associated fat and cholesterol content poses other challenges.

A healthy diet should be the major source of essential minerals but all of the above suggests that the foods we have relied upon for our nutritional minerals are no longer adequate or dependable sources. Therefore, it is a wise alternative to make a complete high-potency supplement of essential minerals a part of any core nutritional supplementation program. Amino acid chelates have proven to be the most effective form for maximum bioavailability since they increase the solubility and stability of these minerals and favor their efficient membrane transport.

(iv) **Antioxidants**. Nutritionists around the world have focused much attention in recent time on the need to prevent the lethal premature oxidation that derails normal cell metabolism. The same oxygen that keeps us alive can have toxic effects in cells. When a bond breaks to split molecules, the two *free radicals* formed are highly reactive species that often combine with oxygen to form other peroxy- and hydroxy- radicals. As we saw in Chapter 5, these unstable indiscriminate 'hotheads' then bombard everything in sight with devastating consequences. For example, if they attack your DNA or RNA, they mess up your genetic code and all the cell metabolism becomes uncontrolled and that can have fatal consequences to the cell and to the body. Almost as many as 100 different diseases, particularly conditions like cancer, alzheimer's, arthritis, atherosclerosis, and many degenerative conditions, have been linked to free radical damage.

The formation of free radicals and subsequent oxidation is favored by environmental toxins, radiation exposure, ultraviolet rays with sunlight exposure, exercise and more forms of oxidative stress, among other things. To neutralize these deadly effects of free radicals and premature oxidation, the body needs antioxidants. This has been given much attention by the media in recent time and most people now think of antioxidants in their food. Much is made of beta carotene in carrots and yellow fruits (like peaches, apricots, mangoes) and lycopenes in fresh garden tomatoes. Many people buy supplements of vitamins A, C and E as well as the mineral selenium for their antioxidant effects. Others exploit the properties of whey protein concentrates that contain precursors for cells to increase glutathione (GSH) production (2). This is an endogenous antioxidant formed only within the cells.

More recently, there has been a focus on another powerful cellular antioxidant called superoxide dismutase (SOD). Scientists at Albion Labs have also formulated a proprietary mineral complex which supplies the building blocks of an effective SOD Precursor System to enhance this major cellular antioxidant. Other potent antioxidants are derived from *Maritime Pine Bark* extract and *Grape Seed* extract, the potency of which is enhanced by "macerating enzymes." Together, these enhance the body's ability to fight off free radicals and then take care of the toxic waste.

(v.) Probiotics (friendly bacteria). Our health depends on the friendly flora strains which live in our intestines. These vital microorganisms decrease fat and cholesterol levels in our blood, help correct yeast overgrowth, and also promote proper elimination, helping to rid the body of toxins. They aid digestion (especially of dairy products), increase mineral absorption and help to protect from infections and several chronic diseases. These good bacteria are believed to be destroyed by antiobiotics, as well as by laxatives, oral contraceptives, carbonated drinks, alcohol, stress and even some digestive aids.

Oral supplements of *bifido bacterium bifidum*, commonly called bifidus, is used to prevent acute diarrhea in young children, to provide healthful bacteria to human adults, and to re-seed intestinal bacteria affected by diarrhea, chemotherapy, advancing age, antibiotics and other causes.   It is the predominant intestinal flora of breast-fed infants. Ingestion of yogurt fermented with bifidus increases the number of bifido bacteria in the stool and suppresses coliform bacteria.

Another similar supplement, *lactobacillus acidophilus* is used for improving lactose tolerance as well as for treating vaginal and urinary tract infections, antibiotic-induced diarrhea, oral candida, irritable and inflammatory bowel disorders, and more. Acidophilus (as it is commonly known) is a native inhabitant of the human gastrointestinal tract and is found in dairy products, especially milk and yogurt. The practice of supplementation with probiotics is essentially safe.

Total flora support however, will only be obtained by using up to twelve *different strains* of friendly bacteria.   Dr. Khem Shahani has developed proprietary processes for stabilizing these strains and making them commercially available. As we mentioned in chapter 6, their potency can be increased by the addition of fructooligosaccharides (FOS).

In summary, as you design your own menu for your personal application of **The Enzyme Diet™ Solution**, here are the **Ten Basic Considerations** to guide your many choices.

1. **Eat Small, Regular and Varied Meals.**
2. **Drink at least Eight Glasses of fluid each day.**
3. **Favor foods with Low Glycemic Index.**
4. **Run away from Fat.**
5. **Eat as many Raw Foods as possible.**
6. **Shop for Health.**
7. **Avoid Crash Diets.**
8. **Practice Responsible Fasting.**
9. **Occasionally Treat Yourself.**
10. **Supplement your Normal Diet.**

With these initial guidelines in mind, you can now go on to design your personal menu and complete **The Enzyme Diet™ Solution**. Following are some recipe suggestions to get started. There are enough ideas to make dinners for two full weeks, complete with nutritional values for calories and more. Then follows some useful suggestions for creating a healthy kitchen. Since you will not always eat at home, we include a number of practical suggestions for eating out. Finally, some tips for snacking are added to round off your complete dietary plan. Remember to hold your daily calorie count at about 1200 calories or more during your active weight loss phase and then at about 1500-2000 during maintenance, depending on your lifestyle.

Recipe Ideas to Suit Your Taste

1.	Pasta with Garlic Chicken, Roasted Peppers and Basil

2 tablespoons olive oil
1 cup chopped onion
2 cloves garlic, minced
1 can no-salt added whole tomatoes, undrained and chopped
1 large green pepper, roasted and peeled
1 large sweet red pepper, roasted and peeled
1 large sweet yellow pepper, roasted and peeled
¼ teaspoon salt
¼ teaspoon freshly ground pepper
8 ounces dry penne (short tubular pasta)
¼ cup thinly sliced fresh basil
¼ cup freshly grated Parmesan cheese
3 large or 4 medium boneless, skinless chicken breast halves
Cook pasta according to package directions, omitting fat and salt.

SAUCE
Heat 1 tablespoon olive oil in large nonstick skillet over medium-low heat. Add chopped onion and 1 clove minced garlic to oil. Cover mixture and cook 10 minutes or until tender, stirring occasionally. Add chopped tomatoes to onion mixture and bring to a boil. Reduce heat and simmer, uncovered, 30 minutes, stirring occasionally.

Cut roasted green, red, and yellow peppers into julienne strips (¼ to ½ inch). Add roasted pepper strips, salt and freshly ground pepper to tomato mixture; cook 3 minutes or until thoroughly heated.

Combine tomato mixture, cooked pasta and basil in a large bowl and toss mixture well.

GARLIC CHICKEN
Remove all visible fat and skin from chicken. Slice chicken into ½ inch strips. Sprinkle ground pepper on chicken strips. Add 1 tablespoon olive oil to non-stick fry pan on medium heat. Add 1 clove minced garlic to oil and cook for 1 minute. Add peppered chicken to garlic and oil mixture. Cook chicken until lightly brown, stirring frequently (about 8 to 10 minutes).

Serve 1 cup pasta mixture onto plate and add 5 to 6 chicken strips, then sprinkle with Parmesan cheese. (Yield: 4 servings)

Nutrition Facts Per Serving
Calories: 328 (20% from Fat)
Protein: 33 g   Fat: 7.3 g (saturated = 2.0 g)
Carbohydrate: 32.6 g

Tips: To increase the fiber content, choose whole grain pasta.

2.	**Feta-Stuffed Chicken over Spinach Salad**

4 (4-ounce) skinless, boneless chicken breast halves
¼ cup dry breadcrumbs
¼ cup crumbled feta cheese with basil and tomato
1 ½ teaspoons butter, melted
3 cups torn spinach
½ cup chopped fresh basil
1 tablespoon balsamic vinegar
1 tablespoon olive oil
1/8 teaspoon freshly ground pepper

Place each chicken breast half between 2 sheets of heavy-duty plastic wrap; flatten to ¼ inch thickness using a meat mallet or rolling pin. Dredge chicken in breadcrumbs. Spoon 1 tablespoon cheese onto each piece of chicken; fold chicken in half.

Place folded breast halves in 8-inch square baking dish coated with cooking spray or ½ tablespoon olive oil. Drizzle melted butter over chicken. Bake, uncovered at 400 degrees for 25 minutes or until chicken is done.

Combine spinach and basil in a bowl; drizzle vinegar and oil. Sprinkle pepper over salad; toss well. Serve chicken over salad. Yield: 4 servings (serving size: 1 chicken breast half and ¾ cup salad)

Nutrition Facts Per Serving:
Calories: 207 (26% from Fat)
Protein: 29.6 g   Fat: 6.2 g (sat 1.9 g)   Carbohydrate: 7.0 g

Try a variation of this dish: **Feta-Stuffed Chicken and Rice**
Serve with 1 cup steamed vegetables and ½ cup brown rice instead of spinach salad.
Nutrition Facts Per Serving
Calories: 312 (20% from Fat)
Protein: 32.1 g   Fat: 7.0 g (sat 2.0 g)   Carbohydrate: 30 g

3.   Teriyaki Chicken and Vegetables

4 (4-ounce) skinless, boneless chicken breast halves
1 tablespoon olive oil
¼ to ½ cup teriyaki sauce
¼ tsp ground ginger
1 clove minced garlic
2 cups shredded or sliced cabbage
2 cups chopped broccoli
2 cups sliced bell peppers
1 cup chopped onions (optional)

Trim excess fat from chicken. Place each chicken breast half between 2 sheets of heavy-duty plastic wrap; flatten to ¼ inch thickness using a meat mallet or rolling pin. Slice chicken into ¾ inch strips. Place strips in bowl with ¼ to ½ cup teriyaki sauce. Ensure that all strips are covered with sauce. Place bowl in refrigerator to marinate for 20 minutes.

Heat 1 tablespoon olive oil in large nonstick skillet over medium to medium-high heat. Add garlic, ginger and onions to oil and cook for 1-2 minutes. Add broccoli, bell peppers and cabbage to mixture and cook for 2-3 minutes stirring frequently. Add chicken strips and teriyaki sauce from bowl to mixture and continue stirring mixture until chicken is thoroughly cooked.

Serve over ½ cup brown rice or wheat noodles and drizzle 1 tablespoon teriyaki sauce over plate of rice (or noodles) and chicken, vegetable mixture. (Yield: 4 servings)

Nutrition Facts Per Serving
Calories: 377 (18.4% from Fat)
Protein: 34.5 g   Fat: 7.7 g (sat 1.5 g)   Carbohydrate: 42.4 g

Try this variation - **Teriyaki Chicken Wrap**
Follow recipe above for preparation. Add ¾ cup chicken, vegetable mixture and ¼ cup rice to center of burrito-size whole-wheat tortilla. Drizzle ½ tablespoon teriyaki sauce over mixture and wrap.

Nutrition Facts per Serving:
Calories: 387 (20% from Fat)
Protein: 27 g   Fat: 8.6 g (sat 2 g)   Carbohydrate: 50 g

4.   Black Bean and Rice Burritos

1 tablespoon Mexican spice blend
1 teaspoon garlic powder
¼ teaspoon ground cumin
1 15-ounce can black beans (undrained)
1 ¾ cups cooked long-grain brown rice (cooked without salt or fat)
6 whole wheat flour tortillas

½ cup shredded reduced-fat sharp Cheddar cheese
¼ cup sliced green onions
¼ to ½ cup salsa
¼ cup nonfat sour cream (optional)
Combine the first 4 ingredients in a medium saucepan and bring to a boil. Reduce heat, and simmer uncovered, 5 minutes, stirring occasionally. Remove from heat and stir in rice.

Spoon about 1/3 cup bean mixture down center of each tortilla. Top with 2 tablespoons cheese, 1 tablespoon green onions, 1 tablespoon salsa and 1 tablespoon sour cream (optional). Roll up and enjoy. Yield: 6 servings

Nutrition Facts Per Serving:
Calories: 332 (15% from fat)
Protein 16.1 g   Fat: 5.7 g (sat 2.1 g)   Carbohydrate 53.9 g

Try this variation: **Chicken, Black Bean and Rice Burrito**
Add 1-2 oz of grilled chicken breast strips. Prepare chicken strips by removing excess fat from two (4 oz) boneless, skinless chicken breast halves. Slice into ½ to 1 inch strips and sprinkle with Mexican spice. Add 2 teaspoons olive oil to non-stick skillet over medium-high heat. Cook chicken strips until golden brown and thoroughly cooked.

Nutrition Facts Per Serving:
Calories 396 (20% from fat)
Protein: 25 g   Fat: 8.9 g (sat 2.7 g)   Carbohydrate: 53.9 g

5.	Beef Burgundy

1 ¼ pounds lean, boneless round steak
2 cloves minced garlic
½ cup diced onions
1 cup burgundy or other dry red wine
½ can reduced-fat, reduced-sodium cream of mushroom soup
½ can beef consommé (undiluted)
3 cups sliced fresh mushrooms

1 ¼ cup pearl onions
1 ½ tablespoons all-purpose flour
1 12-ounce package medium egg noodles, uncooked
¼ cup grated Parmesan cheese
¼ cup nonfat sour cream
Cooking spray or olive oil for coating

Trim fat from steak. Cut steak into 1-inch cubes. Coat an ovenproof Dutch oven with cooking spray or olive oil; place over medium heat until hot. Add steak; cook 9 minutes or until steak is no longer pink. Drain well; set aside. Wipe drippings from Dutch oven with paper towel.

Coat Dutch oven with cooking spray or olive oil; place over medium heat. Add minced garlic and diced onions; sauté 1 minute. Add wine/burgundy, mushroom soup and beef consommé; stir well, and bring to a boil. Return steak to Dutch oven; stir in mushrooms and pearl onions. Remove from heat.

Place flour in a small bowl. Gradually add 1/4 cup water, blending with a wire whisk; add to steak mixture, stirring well. Cover and bake at 350 degrees for 1 ½ hours.

Cook egg noodles according to package directions, omitting salt and fat. Drain noodles well, and place in a large serving bowl. Add Parmesan cheese and sour cream; toss mixture gently to coat. Serve steak mixture over noodle mixture. Yield: 6 servings (serving size: ¾ cup steak mixture and 1 cup noodle mixture)

Nutrition Facts per Serving
Calories 411 (17% from fat)
Protein: 32.8 g   Fat: 7.7 g (sat 2.3 g)   Carbohydrate: 52.5 g

6.	Beef with Broccoli

1 pound lean, boneless top round steak
1 teaspoon coarsely ground black pepper
½ teaspoon vegetable oil
4 cups fresh broccoli florets

½ cup sliced green onions
1 cup sliced & seeded tomatoes
2 cloves minced garlic
1/3 cup dry white wine
½ cup low-sodium soy sauce
4 teaspoons cornstarch
4 cups hot cooked long-grain brown rice (cooked without salt or fat)

Trim fat from steak. Slice steak diagonally across grain into thin strips. Sprinkle black pepper over steak slices. Coat a wok or large nonstick skillet with cooking spray or olive oil; place over medium-high heat until hot. Add peppered steak, and stir-fry 3 minutes. Remove steak from wok; set aside, and keep warm.

Add ¼ teaspoon vegetable oil to wok, and place over medium-high heat until hot. Add green onions, and garlic; stir-fry 1 minute. Add broccoli; stir-fry 3 minutes. Add tomatoes; stir-fry 1 minute.

Combine wine, soy sauce and cornstarch; stir well. Add cornstarch mixture and steak to wok; stir-fry 1 minute or until sauce is thickened and bubbly. Serve over rice. (Yield: 4 servings) each of 1 cup steak & broccoli mixture and 1 cup rice)

Nutrition Facts Per Serving:
Calories: 469 (17% from fat)
Protein: 33.5 g   Fat: 9.4 g (sat 2.9 g)   Carbohydrate: 62.7 g

---

7.   Shrimp Fajitas with Black Beans and Spanish Rice

¾ pound uncooked shrimp
1 Tbsp. olive oil
1 clove minced garlic
3 teaspoons fajita seasoning or Mexican seasoning
½ teaspoon black pepper
2 cups sliced bell peppers (red, green and/or yellow)
1 sliced onion
8 whole wheat or corn tortillas
1 can black beans

FAJITAS
Peel shrimp and place in bowl. Add 2 teaspoons seasoning mix to coat shrimp in seasoning; set aside. Heat 1 tablespoon olive oil in large non-stick skillet over medium-high heat. Add garlic and stir-fry for 1 minute. Add bell peppers, onions, ½ teaspoon fajita seasoning and ½ teaspoon black pepper. Stir-fry for 2 minutes. Add shrimp to skillet and stir-fry until shrimp is pink and thoroughly cooked. Add remaining ½ teaspoon fajita seasoning during last few minutes of cooking.

SPANISH RICE
2 cups cooked rice (cooked without salt or fat)
2 teaspoons olive oil
1/8 teaspoon saffron powder
1/4 cup chopped onion
1/8 cup chopped celery
1/4 cup chopped green pepper
1/8 cup chopped sweet red pepper
1 clove crushed garlic
1/8 cup no-salt added tomato sauce
1/2 teaspoon chili powder
1/4 teaspoon sugar
1/4 teaspoon salt, 4 tbsp. salsa (optional)
1 can (8oz) no-salt added, whole tomatoes, drained and chopped

Heat 1 teaspoon oil in a large nonstick skillet over medium heat. Add rice and saffron; stir-fry 3 minutes. Remove from skillet; set aside and keep warm. Heat remaining 1 teaspoon oil in skillet over medium-high heat. Add onion, celery, green pepper, sweet red pepper and garlic; stir-fry 2 minutes or until tender. Add tomato sauce and remaining ingredients; cook 2 minutes, stirring often. Return rice to skillet and stir-fry until thoroughly heated.

BLACK BEANS
Heat can of black beans in sauce pan as directed on can.

Add ½ cup fajita mixture to each tortilla (2 tortillas per serving). Serve with ½ cup Spanish rice and ½ cup black beans. Add 1 Tbsp salsa to each fajita if desired. (Yield: 4 servings.)

Nutrition Facts Per Serving:
Calories: 505 (15% from fat)
Protein: 29.9 g   Fat: 8.8 g (sat 0.75 g)   Carbohydrates: 76.7 g

---

8. Grilled Portabella Mushroom Sandwich/Balsamic Pasta Salad

MUSHROOM SANDWICH
5 large portabella mushrooms
6 teaspoons balsamic vinegar
2 teaspoons olive oil
½ teaspoon coarsely ground pepper.
5 whole wheat round sandwich rolls (hamburger size)
10 slices provolone cheese (deli-sliced)
2 tomatoes thinly sliced
5 leafs of green-leaf or red-leaf lettuce

Pre-heat oven to 350 degrees.
Remove stems from mushrooms. Mix 2 teaspoons olive oil, 2 teaspoons balsamic vinegar and ½ teaspoon pepper in a small bowl. Add olive oil mixture to non-stick skillet over medium heat. Add mushrooms to skillet stem-side up. Pour remaining balsamic vinegar onto mushroom caps in skillet. Cook each side for 2 minutes and remove pan from heat.

Place whole-wheat buns open face on cookie sheet. Place cooked mushroom caps on 'bottom' buns and cover each with 1 slice of provolone cheese. Place 2nd slice of cheese on top bun. Place cookie sheet in oven and change oven setting to broil. Broil until cheese is melted, then remove from oven and add tomato slices and lettuce.

BALSAMIC PASTA SALAD
1/3 cup balsamic vinegar
3 tablespoons water
1 ½ teaspoons olive oil
¼ teaspoon salt
½ teaspoon pepper
1 large clove garlic, minced
½ cup small broccoli florets

½ cup julienne-sliced carrot, 1/2 cup cauliflower
½ cup julienne-sliced sweet red pepper
4 cups cooked bow tie pasta (cooked without salt or fat)
2 tablespoons thinly sliced fresh basil
¼ cup (1 ounce) grated Asiago, Romano or Parmesan cheese

Combine vinegar, water, olive oil, salt, pepper and garlic in a jar; cover tightly, and shake vigorously. Set aside. (You may also use a blender to blend these ingredients).

Drop broccoli, cauliflower and carrots into a large saucepan of boiling water; cook 30 seconds. Drain. Pour cold water over vegetables and drain.

Combine drained vegetables, red pepper, cooked pasta, basil and cheese in a large bowl. Add vinegar mixture; toss gently. Cover salad and chill. Yield: 5 servings (serving size = 1 cup pasta salad and 1 sandwich).

Nutrition Facts Per Servings:
Calories: 449 (26% from Fat)
Protein: 22 g   Fat: 13 g (sat 5.9 g)   Carbohydrate: 61 g

9.   Glazed Mahi Mahi, Orzo and Fresh Tomato-Squash

GLAZED MAHI-MAHI
3 tablespoons honey
3 tablespoons teriyaki sauce
1 teaspoon peeled, minced ginger root
4 cloves garlic, crushed
4 (4-ounce) mahi-mahi fillets
1 ½ teaspoons olive oil
1 dash salt
¼ teaspoon freshly ground pepper
3 cups cooked orzo (rice-shaped pasta)

Combine honey, teriyaki sauce, ginger root and garlic in a shallow dish; stir well. Place fish in a single layer over mixture in dish, turning to coat.

Cover and marinate in refrigerator for 20 minutes, turning fish once. Remove fish from marinade, reserving the marinade for later.

Heat oil in a nonstick skillet over medium-high heat until hot. Add fish, and cook 6 minutes. Turn fish; sprinkle with salt and pepper. Cook 3 minutes or until fish flakes easily when tested with fork. Remove from skillet; keep warm.

Add reserved marinade to skillet; cook over medium-high heat 1 minute, deglazing skillet by scraping particles that cling to bottom. Spoon glaze over fish. Yield: 4 servings (serving size: 3 oz fish).

TOMATO-SQUASH SALAD
1 large yellow squash diagonally sliced
1 medium zucchini squash diagonally sliced
4 small tomatoes cut into ½-inch thick wedges
1/2 cup vertically sliced purple onion
1/8 cup packed small fresh basil leaves
1/4 cup white wine vinegar
1 ½ teaspoons olive oil
1/8 teaspoon salt
1/8 teaspoon freshly ground pepper
1 clove garlic minced

Arrange squash in a steamer basket over boiling water. Cover and steam 1 minute; drain. Plunge squash into ice water; drain well. Combine tomato wedges, onion and basil in a large bowl; set aside.

Combine vinegar, olive oil, salt, pepper and garlic; stir well. Pour over vegetables; toss gently. Serve at room temperature or chilled. Yield: 4 servings (serving size: 1 cup).

Serve mahi-mahi over orzo, with tomato-squash salad on the side.

Nutrition Facts per Serving:
Calories: 405 (13% from Fat)
Protein: 33.4 g   Fat: 5.6 g (sat 0.9 g)   Carbohydrates: 55 g

| 10. | Barbequed Chicken, Green Beans and Roasted Red Potatoes |

ROASTED RED POTATOES
6 red potatoes
2 Tsp olive oil, or cooking spray
¼ teaspoon salt
½ teaspoon freshly ground pepper
¼ cup grated Romano or Parmesan cheese

Preheat oven to 350 degrees. Wash potatoes and slice into 1 ½ inch cubes. Combine olive oil, salt and ground pepper in small dish. Coat 9 ½ x 13 inch baking pan with cooking spray or olive oil. Spread potatoes in single layer in baking pan. Pour olive oil mixture evenly over potatoes ensuring that they are all coated. Sprinkle cheese over potatoes. Bake 25 to 30 minutes at 350 degrees.

BBQ CHICKEN
4 boneless, skinless chicken breast halves
½ cup barbeque sauce
¼ cup diced purple onion

Combine barbeque sauce and ¼ cup diced onion in shallow dish; stir well. Remove excess fat from chicken and use a fork to poke holes throughout chicken. Place chicken in a single layer over mixture in dish, turning to coat. Cover and marinate in refrigerator for 20 minutes, turning chicken once.

Coat 8 inch baking dish with cooking spray or olive oil. Arrange chicken in single layer in baking dish. Pour excess barbeque sauce on chicken. Bake chicken for 25 to 30 minutes at 350 degrees.

GREEN BEANS
1 pound fresh green beans
½ cup diced purple onion
½ Tsp olive oil
¼ teaspoon salt
¼ teaspoon freshly ground pepper

Wash beans; trim ends, and remove strings. Arrange beans in a vegetable steamer over boiling water. Combine beans with ½ cup diced onions in a bowl. Combine olive oil, salt and pepper; add to bean mixture. Toss gently. Serve warm.

Yield: 4 servings (serving size: 1 chicken breast, 1 cup green beans, 1 cup potatoes)

Nutrition Facts Per Serving:
Calories: 497 Calories (24% from Fat)
Protein: 35 g   Fat: 13.5 g (sat 3.2 g)   Carbohydrate: 58.8 g

11. Teriyaki Salmon, Wild Rice and Asparagus

4 (3 oz) salmon fillets
½ cup teriyaki sauce
1 clove minced garlic
½ teaspoon freshly ground pepper
2 cups cooked wild rice (no fat or salt added)
1 bunch asparagus (approx. 24 spears)

Combine garlic and teriyaki sauce in shallow dish; stir well. Place fish in a single layer over mixture in dish, turning to coat. Cover and marinate in refrigerator for 20 minutes, turning fish once. Remove fish from marinade, reserving marinade for later use.
Wash asparagus and cut ends to leave 4-5 inch tips.

Preheat oven to 350 degrees. Coat 9 x 13 inch baking dish with cooking spray or olive oil. Arrange fish in single layer in baking dish. Arrange asparagus tips around fish in dish. Pour excess marinade over fish and asparagus. Sprinkle ground pepper over fish and asparagus. Bake fish for 20 minutes at 350 degrees. Serve with ½ cup rice. Yield: 4 servings (1 serving = 6 asparagus tips, 1 salmon fillet and ½ cup rice).
Nutrition Facts Per Serving:
Calories: 350 (12% from Fat)
Protein: 33 g   Fat: 4.7 g (0.8 g)   Carbohydrates: 44 g

12. Creamy Chicken Fettuccini

16 oz whole wheat or spinach fettuccine
1 large garlic clove, minced
¼ teaspoon salt
4 boneless, skinless chicken breast halves
3 teaspoons olive oil
2 teaspoons whole wheat flour
1 cup skim milk
¼ tsp black pepper
1 Tbsp grated cheese

Cook fettuccine according to package directions.

Trim excess fat from chicken and slice into 1 inch cubes. Heat 1 teaspoon oil in a large, non-stick skillet. Add garlic; stir fry 1 minute. Add chicken and stir-fry until chicken is no longer pink when pierced at the thickest part (about 5 to 8 minutes). Remove chicken from pan and keep warm. Add remaining two teaspoons of oil to skillet and sprinkle flour over mixture. Stir well. Gradually stir in skim milk; bring to a boil, stirring occasionally until mixture thickens slightly. Return chicken to skillet. Add pepper and salt; mix well. Drain fettuccine, and add it to the skillet, along with the cheese. Toss to mix well. (Yield: 6 servings)

Serve with Spinach and Mushroom Salad (see below).

Nutrition Facts Per Serving:
Calories: 477 (12% From Fat)
Protein: 30.7 g   Fat: 6.3 g (sat 1.3 g)   Carbohydrate: 58.5 g

13. Mussels Steamed in a White Wine Sauce/Spinach Salad

MUSSELS
3 pounds mussels
½ cup coarsely chopped onion
¼ teaspoon thyme

¼ teaspoon freshly ground pepper
1 cup dry white wine
½ cup water
2 teaspoons lemon juice (preferably from freshly squeezed lemons)
¾ cup chopped parsley

Scrub mussels well. With a small sharp knife, cut off hairy brownish 'beards'. Place mussels in a large kettle. Add onion, thyme, pepper, wine, water, lemon juice, and 2 tablespoons parsley. Cover and bring to a boil over high heat. Cook, covered, 5 minutes, until mussels open. Stir once to bring those on the bottom to the top.

Remove mussels with a slotted spoon. Discard any that do not open. Strain juices through a fine sieve lined with cheesecloth to be used as broth. Divide mussels among 4 large soup bowls. Pour hot broth over mussels. Top with remaining parsley. (Yield: 4 servings)

SPINACH MUSHROOM SALAD
½ pound fresh spinach
8 large mushrooms
2 scallions, sliced
4 radishes, sliced
½ c Lemon Mustard Dressing (see instructions below)
1 Tbsp. light soy sauce
Add freshly ground pepper to taste

Wash spinach well. Remove stems and discard. Shake spinach dry and refrigerate while preparing mushrooms. Cut off stem ends of mushrooms and discard. Slice mushrooms. Place spinach leaves and mushrooms in bowl. Add scallions and radishes. Combine Lemon Dressing with soy sauce and pour over salad. Season with salt and pepper.

LEMON MUSTARD DRESSING
Combine the following ingredients and mix well. Makes approx. 1 cup.
½ cup vegetable juice
2 tablespoons red wine vinegar
3 tablespoons lemon juice
1 ½ tablespoons olive oil
1 garlic clove crushed through press

2 teaspoons Dijon mustard
1 tablespoon honey mustard

Serve with 2 slices fresh bread.

Nutrition Facts Per Serving:
Calories: 437 (19% from Fat)
Protein: 32 g   Fat: 9.3 g (sat 1.0 g)   Carbohydrates: 56 g

14.   Healthy Spaghetti

½ pound ground turkey
1 jar (low fat and sodium) spaghetti. Sauce (e.g. Healthy Choice)
4 cups cooked whole wheat noodles
3 cups steamed vegetables of your choice (small broccoli florets, green peppers, onions, mushrooms, zucchini, squash, cabbage)

Wash and slice vegetables of your choice to equal 3 cups. Cook ground turkey in non-stick skillet until brown. Steam vegetables of your choice in a vegetable steamer. Pour sauce into large saucepan; add meat and vegetables to sauce; simmer until hot. Serve over whole-wheat noodles. (Yield: 4 servings)

Serve with Basic Salad
4 cups lettuce (dark green or red leaf)
2 cups spinach leaves
4 cup vegetables (broccoli, grated carrots, diced tomatoes, chopped celery, cucumbers)
Choice of one: 2 avocados, sliced; 4 Tbsp nuts or seeds; or 4 Tbsp grated raw cheese
Low-fat, low-calorie dressing of your choice

Nutrition Facts Per Serving:
Calories: 499 (13% from Fat)
Protein: 35 g   Fat: 7 g (sat 1.5 g)   Carbohydrates: 44 g

NUTRIENT ANALYSIS

The nutritional information provided with each recipe helps you fit these menus into your daily eating plan. The recipes provide both calorie and fat information and we have calculated the percentage of calories from fat for you. Current dietary recommendations encourage eating no more than 30% of calories from fat and cutting this number to 20% is helpful during weight loss. This recommendation applies to the total diet, however - not to individual recipes or foods. The recipes provided in this section contain no more than 30% of calories from fat and many are less than 20% from fat. If you're trying to lose weight, the calorie and fat figures will help you the most.

The suggestions in **Table 11** can help you cut the calories and fat from your favorite recipes. After you've made the adjustments to your favorite recipe, record the new recipe for your new recipe box.

Table 11.   **Low-Fat Ingredient Substitutions**

Needed Ingredient	**Substitute**
Fats and Oils:	
Butter and/or margarine	Margarine made with safflower, soybean, corn oil that are specially processed to ensure that no trans-fatty acids are included. (example: Smart Balance)
Mayonnaise	Nonfat or reduced-calorie mayonnaise
Oil	Safflower, soybean, corn, olive or peanut oil in reduced amount
Salad dressing	Non-fat or oil-free dressing
Shortening	Soybean, corn, canola or peanut oil in amount reduced by one-third
Dairy Products	
Sour cream	Low-fat or nonfat sour cream or yogurt
Whipping cream	Chilled evaporated skimmed milk, whipped
American, Cheddar, Colby, Edam, Swiss	Cheeses with 5 grams of fat or less per ounce
Cottage cheese	Nonfat or 1% low-fat cottage cheese
Cream cheese	Nonfat or light process cream cheese, Neufchatel

	cheese
Ricotta cheese	Nonfat, lite or part-skim ricotta cheese
Milk, whole or 2%	Skim milk, ½% milk or 1% milk
Ice cream	Nonfat or low-fat frozen yogurt, low-fat ice cream, nonfat ice cream sherbet, sorbet

Meats, Poultry, Eggs

Bacon	Canadian bacon, turkey bacon, lean ham
Beef, veal, lamb, pork	Chicken, turkey, or lean cuts of meat trimmed of all visible fat
Ground beef	Extra-lean ground beef, ultra-lean ground beef, ground turkey
Luncheon meat	Skinned, sliced turkey or chicken breast, lean ham
Poultry	Skinned poultry
Tuna packed in oil	Tuna packed in water
Turkey, self-basting	Turkey basted with fat-free broth
Egg, whole	2 egg whites or ¼ cup egg substitute

Miscellaneous

Chocolate, unsweetened	3 tablespoons unsweetened cocoa plus 1 tablespoon margarine (with no trans-fats) per ounce of chocolate
Fudge sauce	Fat-free fudge sauce or chocolate syrup (beware of the sugar content on these substitutes. Some of these will increase sugar to make up for the fat and still have the same number of calories)
Nuts	One-third to one-half less, toasted (toasting the nuts brings out a stronger flavor and you will need less)
Soups, canned	99% fat-free and/or reduced-sodium condensed cream soups

Creating a Healthy Kitchen

If your kitchen isn't set up to promote healthy cooking and healthy lifestyle changes, then your chances of success are greatly decreased. The following guidelines will help you fully implement your Enzyme Diet™ Solution, and thus create a lifestyle of healthy eating. By setting up a healthy kitchen, you will have easy access to the healthiest, most nutritious options. This section contains valuable information for food selection, even if you don't do a lot of cooking at home.

As you read this section, place an "X" in the box beside any step you have already taken. Then, circle the box beside the step you would like to take next. Set goals to complete each step, starting with the one that seems easiest and doing the hardest last.

❏   **Throw Away any *bleached* white flour** you may have and vow never to buy it again. White flour is usually devoid of nutrients, but bleached white flour is even worse!

❏   **Replace Refined, "non-food" items** with healthy foods.

Get Rid of:	Replace with:
White flour - whether bleached or enriched, unbleached flour	Whole wheat pastry flour, oat flour and other whole grain flours
All carbonated beverages & sugary drinks	Water, fresh fruit or vegetable juices
Margarine	Spreads that do not contain trans-fatty acids such as Smart Balance*
	Butter, when cooking
Hydrogenated oils (e.g. shortening, lard, etc.)	
Refined oils	Extra virgin olive oil, cold-pressed oils
Packaged, processed snack-food items	Raisins, nuts, seeds, dried fruit and fresh fruit

❏   **Make a new recipe file box** by following these steps:

○   Purchase several blank or lined 3 x 5 or 4 x 6 index cards, a set of tabbed index cards (with blank tabs) and a new recipe file box.

○   On the tabbed index cards, write your choice of sections (Recommended sections are: Breakfast, Main Dishes, Side Dishes, Snacks and/or Fun Recipes for Kids, Drinks, Shopping Lists.) Place your blank index cards at the front or back of your recipe box, for quick access when you need to record a recipe.

❍   As you try the recipes in **The Enzyme Diet™ Solution** and gather others that fit with **The Enzyme Diet™** Nutrition Plan criteria, record the recipes on cards, then file them in the appropriate section in your file box. If you choose, as you make recipe cards for the earlier recipes, you may want to note that you have done so beside each recipe in the book.

❍   Start new shopping lists on index cards to be placed in your "Shopping Lists" section. Each time you record a new recipe, place the ingredients needed for that recipe on the appropriate shopping list. This will save you a great deal of time because it will eliminate trips back to the store for forgotten items.

❍   Make a 'Shopping List" card** for each place of business where you purchase items (e.g. the 'grocery store', 'health food store', 'bakery' or 'fruit stand.' You may also want to have a card for items you order by mail or telephone on a regular basis. On these cards, record any pertinent information such as prices, address, phone number, ID or membership number, etc.

❍   Once you have enough recipes for a two-week menu (there are 2 weeks of dinner menus provided earlier), you will simply need to keep the items on your newly created shopping lists in stock in order to have all the ingredients you need to prepare your meals and snacks.

    *** The shopping lists in your recipe file will not be lists to take to the store, but rather 'master' shopping lists which you will use in order to check your kitchen's current food supply and make your shopping list of things you will need to purchase.*

❑   **Purchase new cooking tools** that will enable you to use healthy, low-fat cooking methods.

Suggested Cooking Tools:
❍ Spray bottle for water, which can be used in place of oils to keep moisture in foods such as grilled sandwiches, French toast, pancakes

or any food being cooked in a frying pan. The water can be sprayed directly on the food and the pan. It will evaporate and will keep the food from losing too much of its own moisture.

○ Non-stick skillet or wok.

○ Roasting Pan

○ Steamer basket/Rice cooker

○ A good set of sharp knives. Having good knives can save you a tremendous amount of preparation time in slicing vegetables, meats and other food items. It may also be worth your time to take a cooking class that teaches you how to properly use knives.

○ A food processor can save a tremendous amount of time in preparing recipes that call for diced or minced garlic, onion, etc.

○ Citrus juicer

○ Fruit and vegetable juicer. Even very busy people can find time to juice in bulk and freeze juices in zip-lock freezer bags or glass jars when they realize the health benefits of doing so.

○ Strainer/colander with very fine holes for rinsing excess fat from cooked meats such as ground beef. (ground chicken breast is preferable and generally needs no rinsing)

○ Fat separator to separate fat from broths. This item is available at most grocery stores and looks like a measuring cup with a spout at the bottom.

○ Grill basket

Eating Out

Eating out can be problematic when you're trying to lose weight. The problem with eating out is that you can lose control of what goes into your food. Even items that appear to be healthy choices may be full of fat and calories, sometimes enough to ruin or seriously hamper your weight loss efforts. You may be surprised at just how much fat and calories are found in many common fast-food items. **Table 9** gives a selected list.

Table 9   Calories/Fat in Fast-foods/Restaurant Items

Fast-food	Calories	Fat (gm)
16 oz Strawberry Shake	560	16
Big Mac	590	34
Large Fries	540	26
Arby's Giant Roast Beef Sandwich	480	23
Denny's classic burger with cheese	836	53
Denny's Double Decker Burger	1377	92
Arby's Chicken Breast Fillet	540	30
Arby's Grilled Chicken Deluxe	450	22
Arby's Turkey Sub Sandwich	630	37
Arby's Chicken Finger Salad	570	34
McDonald's Chicken McGrill	400	17
Wendy's Chicken Breast Sandwich	430	16
Wendy's Chicken Club Sandwich	470	19
Denny's BBQ Chicken Sandwich	1072	46
Applebee's Veggie Patch Pizza	870	57
Burrito Ultimo, Chicken/Baja Fresh	1070	45
Grilled Veg. Burrito from Baja Fresh	834	37
Arby's Light Grilled Chicken	280	5
Arby's Light Chicken Deluxe	260	5
Arby's Light Roast Turkey Deluxe	260	5
Wendy's Grilled Chicken Sandwich	300	7
Denny's Garden Deluxe Chicken Salad w/ chicken breast	264	11
Applebee's Low-fat Whitefish w/ Mango Salsa	437	9.5
McDonald's Chicken McGrill without mayo	300	6
McDonald's Grilled Chicken Caesar Salad (no dressing)	100	2.5
With the Caesar dressing	250	15.5
TGI Friday's Pacific Coast Chicken	415	8

Don't think we're picking on the fast food industry. Many of the same items at common sit-down restaurants have more than double the calories and fat of those same items at fast-food restaurants.

Even those who are aware that burgers and French fries are high in fat and calories may be shocked at the fat and calorie content of some of the menu choices marketed as "healthy" alternatives to burgers and fries. Just because it's chicken, turkey or a salad doesn't mean it will fit within your diet plan. Let's compare:

The 12.7 ounce Roast Chicken Caesar sandwich from Arby's Market Fresh menu has 820 calories, 38 grams of fat, 9 grams of saturated fat, 140 mg cholesterol, 43 grams protein, 75 grams of carbohydrates, 5 grams of fiber, and 2,160 mg of sodium. This sandwich provides the amount of salt recommended for an entire day and more calories, more fat and more sodium than a McDonald's Big Mac!

The other Market Fresh Sandwiches aren't much better - The Roast Beef and Swiss weighs in at 810 calories and 42 grams of fat, The Roast Turkey and Swiss has 760 calories and 33 grams of fat, and The Roast Ham and Swiss has 730 calories and 34 grams of fat. Although these sandwiches probably supply more fiber - particularly if you choose a whole grain bread - they all have more calories and as much or more fat than the Big Mac.

You should not get the impression that all fast-food and restaurant items are off limits. Most fast-food restaurants offer at least a few healthy alternatives. Take Arby's Light Menu, for example. And many of the menu items marked or described as low-fat, grilled, roasted or heart-healthy items can be a good choice. Include tacos occasionally as a source of fiber.

Smart Tips for Eating Out

These suggestions for eating out will help you avoid the high-calorie, high-fat items that may thwart your weight loss and healthy lifestyle goals.

1- Skip the appetizers. Unless the appetizers are fresh cut fruits and vegetables or salad, it's a good idea to skip them, particularly if you're eating in a restaurant. Some of these dishes have more calories than your meal or may be your entire allotment of calories for the day. Shared or not, these appetizers can add extra padding to your hips and waist. Check out the calorie content of some of the common appetizers below!

Appetizer	Calories
One basket of garlic bread	800
Cheese nachos	810
Buffalo wings with blue cheese dressing	1010
Fried calamari	1040
Stuffed potato skins with sour cream	1260
Fried whole onion with dipping sauce	2130
Cheese fries with ranch dressing	3010

2- Know What You're Ordering. With today's Internet technology, you can access the nutrition information for the menu items at your favorite restaurants at the click of a button. Most restaurants provide nutrition facts on their websites. Make a list of items that fit in the low-fat, low-calorie guidelines and keep them handy. If you can't find the information online, ask for it at your next visit.

3- Ask Questions and ask for dressing and sauces on the side. Ask the server how your food will be prepared. If it doesn't meet your standards for healthy guidelines, ask if it can be prepared differently or if you can make substitutions. For example:

· Ask for steamed vegetables instead of mashed potatoes or French fries.
· Ask for red, tomato-based sauces instead of cream sauces.
· Ask if the item can be grilled or cooked without butter.

Many items are considered healthy, low-fat and low-calorie without the dressing or sauce. Asking for the dressings and sauces on the side helps you control how much fat and calories go into your food.

4- Practice defensive eating. Plan your snacks and meals so that you don't get hungry on the run (e.g. eat a healthy snack before you go out shopping). Avoid fast foods and the mall snacks, lattes and cappuccinos. They can pack on the extra calories without providing much nutrition.

Snack	Calories
Pretzels	370
Small potato fries	460
TCBY regular waffle cone	380
Starbucks café mocha with skim milk	240
Starbucks white chocolate mocha with whole milk	500
McDonald's large French fries	540
Super size	610
KFC large popcorn chicken	620
Pizza Hut personal pan cheese pizza	630
Sbarro spinach & broccoli stuffed pizza	710
Taco Bell mucho grande nachos	1320

5- Avoid fried foods. Look for items that are grilled, broiled and roasted. These items are usually lower in calories and fat, and they are easier to digest.

6- Eat half raw. Starting with a fresh green salad or other raw vegetables will help fill you up and keep you from overeating. You may even want to eat raw vegetables before you go.

7- Watch out for the breads, chips and other items. Many people have a tendency to overeat these items while waiting for their meal. Avoid this by asking your server to bring you only half as much or none at all.

8- Beverages. Order lemon water, water or herb teas and avoid alcohol, mineral water, wine spritzers, soda, coffee and tea. These beverages can add calories and some contain caffeine and carbonation, which can alter digestion and reduce the effectiveness of your body's digestive enzymes.

9- Beware of Dessert. Most of these items are high-calorie and high fat. If the dessert item description uses terms generally associated with a natural disaster (i.e. mudslide, volcano explosion, tornado, blizzard, etc.), it is best to avoid them all-together. If you're tempted by dessert, wait and go out for frozen yogurt or ask for sorbet or fresh fruit.

10- Beware of overgrown serving sizes. Serving sizes in the United States have grown at an exponential rate. Today, most restaurants serve portions that are actually enough for two and sometimes three people. Keep this in mind when you order and remember that you don't have to finish everything on your plate. Ask for a box to take home the extras or share an order with someone else.

Snacking Tips and Ideas

When you're feeling the urge to snack, you must take control and do the healthy thing. Of course, you can include snacks as part of your daily diet but you should eat only limited calorie snacks; eat these only in moderation and try to stick to your schedule. So go ahead and try something different but maintain this healthy approach to snacking.

* Make a shake using The Enzyme Diet™ recipes
* Make banana splits or sundaes using low-fat frozen yogurt.
* Mix frozen yogurt with fresh or frozen fruits and nuts.
* Stir ¼ cup fresh, chilled (almost frozen) orange juice into ¾ cup vanilla yogurt.
* Make frozen juice pops with fresh fruit juice. For variety mix in a little pureed fruit before freezing.
* Freeze fruits (e.g. bananas, strawberries, mango, peaches) for a tasty treat.
* Eat nuts and seeds with raw carrot or celery sticks
* Top celery with raw nut butter
* Dip vegetables (mushrooms, bell peppers, jicama, celery, carrots, sliced yams, etc.).
* Snack on fresh fruits (all varieties, but especially fruits with higher fiber content - e.g. berries and apples)
* Make air-popped popcorn
* Top whole wheat crackers with reduced-fat cheese
* Spread whole grain breads or whole-grain crackers with organic honey or 100% fruit jelly

Suggested snacks to keep around
- Sunflower seeds
- almonds
- whole grain crackers
- cut vegetables and dip
- apples and other easy to eat fruit
- pita bread and hummus
- homemade Popsicle's
- low fat cool whip/whip cream and frozen fruit
- If you must have something chocolate, try fudgsicles (~140 cals)

Tips for controlling cravings and overeating.

· Eat a small piece of food that is high in protein about 20 minutes before lunch and before dinner, such as a piece of reduced-fat cheese or slice of turkey.

· Brush your teeth right after you finish eating. You'll be less likely to snack or eat sweet stuff because there are very few foods that taste good with toothpaste.

· If there are specific foods that you just can't resist (chocolate, Oreos, potato chips, etc), don't keep them in the house. And don't use other family members as an excuse to keep these around. If they love you and support you, they'll be ok with not having those snack foods around anyway.

· Remember that you don't have to finish everything on your plate, even if you're eating out.

· If you're craving something, you may be dehydrated. Drink a glass of lemon water and wait 10 minutes. Find something to do during the 10 minutes. If you're still hungry or craving a specific food after that, go ahead and eat it. It's not worth torturing yourself if the craving is real.

Now that you have devised your own menu, it's time to **Determine your Exercise Level**.

Chapter 9

DETERMINE
YOUR EXERCISE LEVEL
Work It Off - Keep It Off

You would have noticed throughout the book that there has been consistent references to physical activity. After all, exercise is a distinct parameter in the *calorie (energy) balance equation*. But we have waited this long to deal with the subject of exercise in detail for at least three very good reasons.

First, every responsible diet program has always included the role of exercise and this is not by itself a *distinctive* feature of this program. Clearly, a sedentary lifestyle is totally inconsistent with any serious attempt to lose weight and moreso, to keep it off. Some diet programs give but lip service to this valuable lifestyle habit. However, to focus on health as the major consideration of weight, makes exercise a central concern. Exercise will make you look better and feel better, and it will add life to your years and probably years to your life too. It is therefore a critical component of **The Enzyme Diet™ Solution.**

Secondly, by waiting until now to deal with the subject of exercise, we put it in its proper place. Contrary to popular opinion, recent research findings strongly indicate that although any increase in your level of activity will certainly burn up more calories, the net impact over the relatively short weight loss period (typically 12 to 24 weeks or so) is relatively small. But if you really want to *maintain* your new weight over the long haul, exercise must be a major contributing factor. For example, just a brisk walk for half an hour a day, consistently throughout the year, would burn enough calories to equal 20 pounds of fat per year. In a word, exercise is much more important for Phase II maintenance than for Phase I when you're actively trying to lose weight. Nevertheless, it makes consummate sense to begin this new lifestyle pattern as soon as you begin to address your weight issue. That cannot be overstated. The one behavior that correlates best with maintaining weight loss is burning more than 2000 calories per week (1). That's about 300 calories a day. To put this in context, a person weighing 150 pounds walking for 30 minutes (about 1.5 miles or 2.5 kilometers) burns about 200 calories. That's clearly do-able on a daily basis and would be most enjoyable. Weight management is, above all, a life long concern.

The third reason for waiting until now to address this issue in detail is that you may be one of those for whom the mere mention of the word 'exercise' is demotivating and threatening. It may not be your favorite subject, for you're not predisposed to the demands you imagine it imposes. You may think that it's painful, it's boring and you just don't have the time. You may even have memories of sore muscles, useless and expensive gym memberships, or exaggerated mail order gimmicks that you've tried. You've tried and failed. It's not in your genes, and in any case, it's too late now. Even then, with all the confusion and misinformation, you hardly know where to begin.

But you need not fear. Those feelings are universal. All the joggers you see in the parks had the same initial struggles. Ask the receptionist at the gym and you would learn that lots of people show up there with good intentions and leave with them. However, there is a way to exercise that is so effective and takes so little time, that you would be amazed. That's what you are about to learn. It's an attractive component of **The Enzyme Diet™ Solution**.

Before we describe a specific program, let's look at exercise in general, for there are some important distinctions to be made.

The Value of Exercise

Back in the 1980's there seemed to be a fitness revolution. Baby boomers had just discovered aerobics and jogging was in. The annual marathons ballooned in size. Work out videos were among the hottest selling items on television and daily programs kept homemakers hopping every morning. But the fad has been waning in the general public and American lifestyles are becoming more sedentary. The US Surgeon

General's 1996 *Report on Physical Activity and Health* pointed out that more than 60 percent of adults did not participate in even moderate physical activity on a daily basis and one out of every four people was completely inactive (2). Another earlier study estimated that over 92 percent of the population was physically unfit (3).

Many studies have demonstrated that physical fitness can generate remarkable health benefits. It can reduce your chances of contracting an unhealthy condition in the first place (it is **proactive**); if you already have some chronic illness, it will support your healing and help you cope (it is **therapeutic**); and thirdly, it will delay the progression and improve your prognosis (it is **rehabilitative**).

The largest fitness study ever conducted was reported in the *Journal of the American Medical Association* in 1989 (4). It measured the fitness levels of 13,344 men and women and then closely monitored them for eight years. They found death rates were much lower for those people who were more physically fit. The study concluded,

"Higher levels of physical fitness were beneficial, even in subjects with other risk factors such as high blood pressure, elevated cholesterol, cigarette smoking and a family history of heart disease ... Unfit people without any risk factors had a higher risk of dying than fit people with all the major risk factors."

The value of exercise can hardly be overstated. It is effective prevention and treatment of heart disease. Many people have avoided cigarette smoking because they recognize the dangers of heart disease and cancer. But did you know that **the risk of getting heart disease and cancer is even greater for sedentary overweight individuals than for those who smoke** (2)?

Regular exercise is an essential factor in the treatment of elevated cholesterol. It favors the good HDL cholesterol and combined with a low fat diet, it reduces the bad LDL cholesterol. It increases collateral circulation to the all important coronary arteries. Exercise has been shown to lower the risk of colon cancer and breast cancer. All the reasons are not yet clear but the benefits certainly are. Exercise helps to increase bone mass and helps prevent osteoporosis in later life. It even helps reverse that trend in post menopausal women. Active people are less likely to develop adult onset, non-insulin dependent diabetes. And there's more. Exercise reduces low back pain, some headaches and even digestive problems. Studies show that as much as 80 percent of all low back pain is due to weak abdominal muscles.

No question about it, **moderate exercise** stands right up there with **adequate nutrition** and **quitting smoking** as the top three healthy lifestyle interventions that anyone can make to improve both the quality and quantity of life.

ॐ

What You Stand to Gain

As part of **The Enzyme Diet™ Solution** for effective weight loss, there are definitive benefits to be derived from the increased physical activity as part of your new lifestyle.

First, there is the weight loss itself. You recall from Chapter 3 that each pound of fat on the body represents 3500 calories in storage. There is no getting around this: *fat is energy on location, exercise is energy in motion.* In all other areas of life, what you don't use, you lose; but in the case of calories and energy, what you don't use, you gain. So exercise shifts the balance in favor of a slimmer, fitter you.

Secondly, exercise spares your lean muscle mass. To put it in simple terms, when the body uses energy it utilizes first the energy stored in muscle as glycogen. After this is depleted, then it burns either protein or fat. Slow aerobic exercise like walking, favors burning fat in the short term. The longer term strategy would be to build more muscle through resistance exercise.

Thirdly, with increased lean muscle mass, your metabolic rate is maintained. Recall again from Chapter 3 that you could calculate your metabolic rate since each pound of lean muscle mass burns typically 14 calories per day. This is a critical consideration for your goal is to lose fat, not lean mass. We saw earlier the problem of yo-yo dieting was related to the slowing of metabolism with weight loss as the body shifted to a 'starvation' mode. A key factor then in keeping weight off is to retain lean mass and maintain your metabolic rate. That's where exercise makes the difference.

Fourthly, exercise will make you feel better. It will relax your mind and reduce the stress and tension in your life. Nature rewards those who indulge this healthy lifestyle habit by secreting endogenous hormones which act like morphine in the brain to give you a natural high that could become addictive. That's why some fitness buffs jog in extreme weather conditions. Those who exercise in the early morning, tend to arrive at the office on a high that can sometimes be contagious and last throughout the day. It seems to enhance a positive mental outlook and that never hurts.

Next is the benefit to your personal self image. Exercise has a way of making you feel so much better about yourself. You sense being in control. You have high self esteem because you are disciplined and responsible. It's your new way of life. You value and love yourself more when you're doing what's right for you.

Finally - and for too many, most importantly - you'll look better. When you go on a diet, most people would concede that they are actually trying to change the shape of their body. That protruding abdomen, flabby arms and thighs, sagging buttocks and hips do not look good in the mirror or on the beach. Exercise is the only alternative to complement dieting to alter the size, thickness, contours etc, of the body parts you carry around. But whether you want most to feel better or to look better, the prescription to increase your physical activity is still the same.

Exercise delivers!

Different Types of Exercise

The Surgeon General's Report was correct in advocating both "moderate activity" *and* "resistance exercise". The joggers, swimmers, aerobics class teachers and work out video promoters are all strong on the *cardiovascular type of exercise*. That's the "moderate activity." On the other hand, personal trainers, gym instructors and body builders are so much into building muscle, they tend to focus on *strength and resistance training*. That's the other major type of exercise.

The benefits of **cardiovascular (aerobic) exercise** have been highly publicized. Yet, the aerobic craze has produced a great deal of misinformation and faulty programs. Common side effects of improperly performed aerobic exercise include muscle loss, organ damage and eating disorders. There is also an increased risk of injury when participating in aerobic activities.

These problems most often stem from misuse. Most people do cardiovascular exercise to burn fat. However, they often exercise at a much higher level than necessary, which makes the body burn calories from carbohydrates, not fat.

People who do aerobic exercise to lose body fat may see initial results, and, to progress, some think they must continue to exercise longer or harder. However, just adding more time or intensity only increases the incidence of injuries and still does not burn fat. Thus, intense cardiovascular exercise has been linked to degeneration of the joints, especially the back, knees and hips; to states of depression; and to anorexia, bulimia and other obsessive psychological problems.

"*This is one of the most important areas as far as exercise education is concerned,*" says exercise physiologist, Paul Robbins. "*We need to teach individuals how to derive benefit from aerobics without overdoing it. Interval training, which changes from high to low intensity is the most productive and safe way to train.*"

That is true. The bottom line is that cardiovascular (aerobic) exercise is highly desirable, but it must be done safely and wisely.

The other major type of exercise, strength **resistance** training, also offers benefits for every individual. In his book, *Strength Fitness*, Wayne Westcott states, "*Sensible strength training can benefit just about everyone with regard to physical capacity, metabolic function, athletic power, injury prevention and physical appearance ... Most men and women have no idea that unless they perform regular strength exercise they lose approximately five pounds of muscle every ten years. Neither do they understand that this steady loss of muscle is largely responsible for lowering their metabolic rate by 5 percent every decade.*" (5)

Strength training has been proven to increase basal (resting) metabolic rate so more calories are burned even when you're not exercising. It decreases the percentage of body fat and improves the obvious shape of the body as muscles take on definition and fat pads are eliminated. This type of exercise can also provide cardiovascular benefits and boosts energy levels. It can reduce low back pain by strengthening abdominal muscles and improving posture. Resistance exercises also provide added protection against osteoporosis and enhances overall health and well being.

One of the greatest benefits is the "triple" effect on calorie burning that comes from strength training. First, strength training burns calories during the workout. Then, more calories are burned when the muscles are recuperating and rebuilding during the 24 hours following a workout. Third, strength training produces more muscle tissue; and since muscle tissue requires more calories, your metabolism is higher even when you are resting. With strength training your body burns more calories even while you're sleeping.

Strength training results in an increase of *lean* muscle, ideally resulting in the hour-glass shape for women and the V-taper shape for men. This is ultimately what people want to accomplish when they diet, but it is impossible to do it through dieting alone.

⁓   A Sensible 1-2-3 Routine   ⁓

How would you like to be able to achieve the many benefits of cardiovascular exercise and strength training in as little as three hours a week, exercising in your own home? You can. You don't need fancy gadgets or expensive equipment. As an integral part of **The Enzyme Diet™ Solution**, it's again a routine **As Simple as 1-2-3:**

1. **Do moderate AEROBIC EXERCISE for 30 minutes on each of 3 days a week (Mon - Wed - Fri).**

2. **Do a simple RESISTANCE TRAINING workout for 30 minutes on each of the other 3 days (Tues - Thur - Sat).**

3. **Use a DAILY SUPPLEMENT to increase your fat burning potential.**

This simple workout program can readily be adapted to fit your present fitness level, in order to help you achieve your fitness goals. Whether you are just starting a fitness program or are already active, this program will work for you. It's a proven program that has demonstrated high effectiveness and compliance. In other words, those who begin this program, quickly see results and find they can stick with the program for long term benefits. Exercising has never been easier or more healthful. When all 1-2-3 routines are utilized together, there is no other strength training or cardiovascular plan that can produce the kind of results this can, in such a short period of time.

Now, let's look at each of the three basic routines in turn.

1. Safe Aerobics

For years, the positive aspects of cardiovascular exercise have been recognized, yet many people abuse this type of exercise. Apparently, most of us don't fully understand how to get the benefits we desire from cardiovascular exercise.

Most people who choose to do cardiovascular exercise have one primary goal and that is to lose weight, which means they need to burn fat. The problem is that most people maintain a heart rate that is much too high during their work out. As a result, they burn more carbohydrates than fat. Others are exercising at a heart rate that is too low, so they are not burning enough calories and are not able to increase their metabolism. Discouraged, yet determined to get results, many exercisers often increase the length of time they exercise or the exercise intensity. The result has been a higher incidence of injury and unhealthy side effects.

Because of recent research, we recommend interval training as the most effective way to do cardiovascular exercise. Interval training is an effective exercise technique that varies the intensity of your workout both during the workout and throughout the week. This approach will yield the results that people have been looking for from this type of exercise.

During an interval workout you alternate the time spent at a low heart rate (or low-intensity, fat-burning zone) and the time spent at a higher heart rate, which is your high-intensity, calorie-burning zone that effectively raises your metabolism. It is also important to alternate your workouts throughout the week and allow for proper recovery. To accomplish this you rotate low, medium and high-intensity workouts during the week.

Calculate Your "Target Heart Rate"

The most effective way to do cardiovascular exercise is to keep the heart rate below what is known as your "target heart rate". To figure your target heart rate, subtract your age from 220. That figure is then your maximum heart rate. For example, if you are 40 years old, your maximum (target) would be 220 - 40 = 180 beats per minute.

To stay in the "safe zone", where the body burns equal amounts of fat and carbohydrates, the heart rate must be kept much lower while doing cardiovascular exercise. The target rate at which you will burn half carbohydrates and half fat is 60 to 65 percent (or lower) of your maximum heart rate. Anytime exercise is performed at a higher heart rate, less fat is burned while more carbohydrates are used to fuel the body. When exercising at 60 percent, you should be able to carry on a conversation with another individual. This is your zone 1, recovery or "fat-burning" zone.

Initial target heart rate   =   60%   x   (220 - your age)

Again, if you are 40, your initial target rate would be 60 percent of (220-40) which is 108 beats per minute.

The next exercise zone is the "anaerobic threshold". This zone is at approximately 80 to 85 percent of your maximum heart rate. In this zone you are utilizing primarily carbohydrates for fuel, but you are increasing the number of calories burned and increasing your cardiovascular endurance.

The third zone is the Peak Training Zone. The peak zone is approximately 85 to 90 percent of your maximum heart rate. Training in this zone will help increase metabolism. However, this zone should be used only after you have developed a strong base fitness level.

Table 10

Calories Burned in 30 minutes									
Activity	Your Weight (LBS)								
	100	125	150	175	200	250	275	300	350
Aerobic Dancing	182	218	254	290	326	398	434	470	542
Bicycling (12mph)	170	200	230	260	290	350	380	410	470
Golf (Walking)	85	106	127	148	169	211	232	253	295
Jogging (10min/mile)	210	250	290	330	370	450	490	530	610
Racquetball	190	228	266	304	342	418	456	494	570
Skiing (CrossCtry)	200	242	284	326	368	452	494	536	620
Stair Climbing	220	266	312	358	404	496	542	588	680
Swimming (40yds/min)	150	180	210	240	270	330	360	390	450
Walking	135	163	191	219	247	303	331	359	415
Tennis (Singles)	140	170	200	230	260	320	350	380	440

Be active, not intense. Remember, your goal when doing cardiovascular exercise is to be active and to keep your body moving. It's not to increase strength. Because you will be performing cardiovascular exercises on the days when your muscles should be resting from your strength-training workouts, you shouldn't add heavy weights or other kinds of resistance to your cardiovascular routines. High intensity cardiovascular aerobics, such as step aerobics, don't allow the muscles to recuperate like they need to. Find an aerobic activity that is relaxing and fun!

Increase intensity slowly. Have fun, yes. But you won't get away that easy. Your body has an amazing physiology and as you do more exercise, it will adapt to allow you to burn more fat and work at a higher level. Therefore, you must continue to gradually increase your intensity as you progress. If you continue to exercise at the same intensity, you will not see the best results. Keeping an exercise diary is a wise practice - it pays dividends.

☙

2. Strength Training

There are many ways to approach strength training. The most popular techniques are not necessarily the best. We suggest you throw out any preconceived ideas of what is the right way to perform resistance exercises, because most often, what people do and what the research shows are two different things.

Appendix 'C' contains descriptions for a dozen simple exercise routines that you can do at home as part of your strength (resistance) training workout.

To maintain consistent results from your strength training, the amount of time you work out does not need to increase. Instead, you will increase the amount of resistance (weight) if necessary. You may eventually want to add dumbbells or barbells to your home workout equipment; however, some people simply use household objects such as soup cans or plastic milk jugs filled with water to increase the resistance.

After thorough research, we strongly recommend a technique that has proven to be the most effective and safest way to perform strength training exercises. This technique involves more muscle fiber than other methods, which means more dramatic results can be attained in less exercise time. It's known as **Super-Slow**. The following guidelines will help you understand how to do Super-Slow correctly and will illustrate how Super-Slow differs from traditional strength training techniques.

It's simple, not complicated. The Super-Slow routine is very simple. It focuses on the major muscle groups, including exercises that are biomechanically correct, or in other words, exercises that comply with and encourage the body's normal range of movement.

It's slow, not fast. Super-Slow is performed using a very slow movement. The most immediate and dramatic results are achieved when exercises are performed using a 7/7 count. In other words, the hard part of the exercise (lifting the weight up, or the positive movement) should take seven seconds, and the easy part (returning the weight back down, the negative movement) should take seven seconds. Use this 7/7 count whether you are lifting weights, or whether your body (and gravity!) are supplying the resistance, as in many of the exercises we recommend.

Often, in traditional weight lifting programs, a count of two seconds up and four seconds down is used. However, the slower, more controlled movements of Super-Slow have been proven to be safer and more effective, providing at least 59 percent better strength gains.

It's smooth, not jerky. Perform exercises with a smooth, flowing movement, being careful not to stop and rest at the top or bottom. Instead, keep the exercise going. It is also important to breath consistently and constantly with each repetition. Use a Lamaze-type breathing style - breathing in and out of your mouth with deep, even breaths.

It's brief, not long. A typical workout session should last only 20-30 minutes. There are two advantages to keeping your workouts short. First, you will find it easier to consistently schedule time to work out. Second, it actually does your body more harm than good to work out for long periods of time. If you exercise more than 45 minutes to an hour, the body begins to produce increased amounts of cortisol, the hormone that "eats" the muscle you are trying to create.

It's focused, not haphazard. Although brief, your workout should be challenging and intense. One set of focused, quality repetitions can accomplish much more than multiple sets using a haphazard approach. To make each repetition a "quality" repetition; keep your breathing consistent and focus on the particular muscle you are working. Always maintain good form and above all, make sure you perform each exercise to complete muscle fatigue. Muscle fatigue means to the point that it is impossible to do another repetition in good form. Completely fatiguing the muscle is necessary in order to see results. The exciting thing about this kind of exercise is that usually, by the very next session, you will see improvement and you will be able to perform more repetitions or will need to increase the resistance for that exercise in order to reach fatigue.

It's every other day, not daily. While many people think it is beneficial to do strength training daily, this isn't true. When you exercise using resistance, you break the muscle fibers down, and they need a day to rest and to rebuild themselves. This is how your strength increases, by breaking those fibers down and then allowing them to recover.

Some people think they should work out sets of muscles at a time - leg muscles one day and arms the next, for example. This is not the case. The body is a dynamic machine that functions best when all parts are working synergistically. Rather than working different muscle groups each day, as some programs suggest, you will find that the body works best when you exercise all muscles of the body to fatigue on the same day, and then allow them to rest for a day.

This is perhaps one of the most important of these recommendations. Remember the **1-2-3** program. First, perform the resistance exercises every other day, i.e. Monday, Wednesday and Friday, or Tuesday, Thursday and Saturday. Second, on the three "off-days" do cardiovascular exercise. Then, one day a week, rest completely from any exercise. We'll come to the third component shortly.

Here are some final **SUMMARY TIPS** to make this exercise program convenient and effective for you:

1. **Stretch to warm up** before any serious exertion. Extend, flex and rotate all major joints in your limbs, torso and neck.
2. **Always breathe consistently** during the full movement of each repetition. Use your rib cage.
3. **Perform each exercise using the 7/7 count** (seven seconds up and seven seconds down).
4. **Perform each exercise to failure** - or in other words for as many repetitions as you can with proper form, up to 15 repetitions. After you can do 15 repetitions with good form using the 7/7 count, add resistance. (The "crunches" exercise is the only exception to the 15-rep rule. Do as many crunches as you can each workout.)
5. **Do this workout three days a week** on alternating days. This exercise routine can be done even when traveling or on vacation.
6. **Add cardiovascular exercise to your strength training regimen** by doing at least 20 to 30 minutes of properly performed aerobics three times a week.
7. **Use a workout chart to track** your progress.
8. **Be consistent with your workouts**. Make your health a priority by doing whatever it takes to arrange your schedule so you can include time to exercise.
9. **Make sure to get adequate sleep**. It is recuperative.
10. **Avoid cold chills** immediately after workout, especially in winter.

With this exercise program, you won't be doing daily, long, complicated, haphazard workouts of fast, jerky exercises. Instead, you will be following a simple routine of cardiovascular workouts and slow, smooth exercises in brief, but intense, 20-minute sessions, alternating every other day. Performing safe aerobic routines and the suggested Super Slow exercises properly will yield exciting results in terms of maintaining weight loss, while affording greater fitness, shapeliness, health and vitality.

There are obviously other types of strength training besides Super-Slow. If you are training for a specific purpose or sport, Super-Slow may not be the best type of training for you. If you are into football, for example, you need to train more for power and explosiveness. That calls for different conditioning exercises and Super-Slow will not get you there. But if weight loss is your prime concern, Super-Slow is clearly the way to go.

3. Increase the Fat-Burning Potential

As a result of a recent discovery, we recommend that you take a lipase/chromium supplement to further increase the fat-burning benefit of cardiovascular exercise.

Why?

This breakthrough came as a result of a recent study in which an exercise physiologist tested 45 people with the same special machine mentioned in Chapter 3, called a *metabolic cart*. The machine measures Respiratory Exchange Ratio (RER) which indicates whether the body is burning fat or carbohydrates during exercise. The RER test indicated that most people had to stay at a relatively low heart rate in order to burn fat.

However, when those same people were given a product containing specific fat digesters and other supporting nutrients, within 30 minutes they were able to exercise at a higher heart rate and still burn mostly fat. By aiding the body's fat digesting capabilities and optimizing insulin function, exercisers can achieve the benefits they have wanted from aerobics. This amazing breakthrough could impact the exercise industry worldwide and could give aerobics the facelift it has needed to be able to consistently deliver results.

Lipase for fat digestion

The problem is that most of the fat we eat is from poor sources. It isn't raw, it lacks enzymes and therefore cannot be readily digested. As we saw in Chapter 4, the enzyme lipase is necessary to break fat down so it can be used for energy. Without lipase, fat is stored or it is only partially broken down, meaning it can then circulate in the bloodstream and cling to the walls of the arteries. Lipase is not present in most diets. So no predigestion takes place. The pancreas then has an additional burden. Therefore, supplementing with this important enzyme is vital to health.

Too much sugar

Not only that, but we also have the problem of sugar and insulin control. As we saw in Chapter 3, eating *too much sugar* tends to create mood swings, cravings and headaches, and can lead to hypoglycemic or diabetic tendencies. Sugar can interfere with consistent production of insulin, the hormone that the body secretes to help control hunger, and regulate energy, fat burning and muscle building. Animal studies have shown that a diet high in simple sugars also produces insulin resistance and changes in the liver enzymes regulating glucose metabolism. Insulin surges can cause people to eat 60 to 70 percent more at the following meal. Although relatively low in calories, beware when it comes to *"fat-free"* - but high sugar - cookies, cakes and other snacks!

Recent research (7) has also shown that eating a diet high in simple sugars can cause the liver to produce more triglycerides, which raises blood triglycerides (a known risk factor for heart disease). This same research has shown a possible link between increased triglycerides and diabetes.

Chromium - Essential for Insulin Function

These problems are compounded because an estimated *90 percent of Americans fail to meet the daily requirements for the mineral chromium* (8). Chromium ensures that insulin works efficiently and plays an essential role in carbohydrate and fat metabolism (9). Chromium deficiency causes fatigue, leads to excess fat production, and is a contributor to diabetes. This deficiency, coupled with the abuse of fat and sugars, may be linked to the lack of energy, mood swings and obesity that so many people experience.

Much has been publicized about chromium, but the chromium that is often promoted is not in the best form.   Chromium picolinate, which is chromium bound to picolinic acid, has been shown to cause liver toxicity and has also been linked to chromosomel damage in animals (10). However, Lipo-chromizyme™ (Chrome ZME™ in Canada) is a one-of-a-kind supplement developed by the same formulation team at Infinity2 to address these needs.   It includes the patented amino acid chelate, Chromium Chelavite®, which is a highly bioavailable and safe form of chromium.   It also includes active lipase for digesting fat, allowing the body to use more fat stores.   Naturally, it also utilizes the innovative CAeDS® delivery system, the only nutrient delivery system of its kind in the world.

With such amazing credentials, Lipo-chromizyme™ is strongly recommended for anyone trying to reduce body fat or stabilize conditions of blood sugar imbalance.   It is a perfect complement to cardiovascular workouts and strength training to complete your **1-2-3 Enzyme Diet™ Exercise Program.**

You will be pleased to find how easily and quickly you are able to see and feel results as you follow this simple exercise program.   The change in your current activity level need not be dramatic.   As stated in the 1996 Surgeon General's Report, "*modest increases in physical activity are likely to be more achievable and sustainable for sedentary people than are more drastic changes, and it is sedentary people who are at greatest risk for poor health related to inactivity.*"   Overall, the report emphasizes the importance of "*activity of at least moderate amount on a regular basis* (2)."

With such a simple **1-2-3** program at your disposal and in your own home, don't wait another day to begin your renewal and rejuvenation, and to start claiming the health benefits you deserve.   You will also look better and feel better as you take complete advantage of **The Enzyme Diet™ Solution.**

You will indeed discover an amazing, new, wonderful YOU!

☙ *Chapter 10* ☙

DISCOVER YOURSELF
Enjoy Life. Enjoy The New You!

Body weight is an intensely personal thing. There's no escaping it. It greets you every morning in the bathroom mirror, it follows you throughout the day by the reflections in the eyes of everyone you meet and it whispers a 'good night' benediction as you put out the vanity light. It's your second face.

After applying **The Enzyme Diet™ Solution**, you will discover that it is indeed possible to lose weight effectively. You will come to realize how much better you look, how much better you feel, and most importantly, how much healthier you are. Whether you lose ten, twenty, thirty … pounds, or much more than that, you'll probably wonder how you ever got that way, and why you even let it slip that far. But *'it's always better late than never'*.

Your appearance will still speak volumes. But then, before you open your mouth publicly, your brighter countenance will communicate a different message. As you speak, your lighter frame will project credibility and more confidence. And after you've gone from each encounter, your new silhouette will provide a personal echo to impress upon the minds of others, a new indelible identity that will resonate with self control.

And that's the key … self control.

There is no substitute for such a disciplined lifestyle. But that cannot be taught or imposed. It is a product of your primary values and subsequent choices. **The Enzyme Diet™ Solution** is only a reward for those earnest seekers who identify their real weight problem and are in search of a practical solution. You must first have a genuine desire to lose weight - especially for the health of it. Then you can make the commitment to follow through, to make the personal application, by sensible dieting as we have outlined and by moderate physical activity as indicated.

If you have the will, then this is the way.

$$\approx$$

Healthy Mind. Healthy Body.

This book has focused on the body much more than on the mind. We have emphasized **reality therapy** - not some kind of hypnosis. We have explored the issues of physiology and biology rather than addressing the challenges of psychology as that applies to weight management in general terms. All that was by design and not by default. **The Enzyme Diet™ Solution** is primarily a biological solution. You cannot wish or will your unwanted pounds away. Those cells of adipose tissue and that triglyceride mass are all real substance - not a figment of anyone's imagination. In fact, all your cells have real needs and they know nothing of hype and advertising. They do not respond to suggestion or deception.

But your mind still matters. Your body is to a large extent, a reflection of your lifestyle and behavior. That, in turn, is a manifestation of your thoughts. As you learned in high school Latin class or Philosophy 101: *cognito ergo sum* - 'I think, therefore I am.' Thought is all you need to authenticate your existence. It is truly all you need to celebrate your identity. If 'cognition' focuses the awareness of your thought and therefore the awareness of yourself, then 'cogitation' and 'consideration' illuminate the content of that thought and thereby the content of your life. It has been wisely postulated by some of the greatest minds that,

> *'What you think, you look.*
> *What you think, you do.*
> *What you think, you are.'* (1)

Your thought life is in a sense, your real life. As an emotional thermostat, it regulates the temperature and tone of your existence. It sets limits to your common experience since you can only appreciate what you truly understand. It initiates the creative expression of life because everything you do reflects a thought going on inside your head. As a thermometer, your perception is a reliable gauge of your true quality of life. Your first awareness is of yourself, then you reflect and project to others and the world around you.

And what does all this mean? You ask.

It means everything, in personal terms. It is hard to perceive an image of yourself, independent of your visible, tangible space-occupying body mass. It's no wonder then that overweight and obesity tend to negatively impact one's self-image and social confidence. In this life, you are confined to your one and only *corpus*. You have to deal with that - it's all you've got. It was Napoleon Hill who said '*Whatever the mind of man can conceive and believe, it can achieve.*'(2)   However, it is also wise to realize that your body can only achieve what your mind can conceive, and that you must believe.

How about you? What do you conceive? What is your self image? What is your body image? How do these two images relate?

Your answers to such questions define and will go a long way to determine your future weight.

All things considered, it could be worse. There is a common *cycle* of negative thinking and irresponsible behavior. It goes something like this. Ineffective weight management by those challenged in this area, for whatever reason, often leads to poor self-esteem. That in turn leads to indifference, resignation and a tendency to isolation. Then eating becomes a mood regulator, a coping mechanism or an assertive impulse - a form of 'acting out.' That increases caloric input which is stored as more unwanted fat. Increasing weight then makes physical activity more burdensome. So the tendency is to exercise less. That again becomes more counter-productive. Feelings of guilt and defeat then increase dependence on food as a type of self indulgence and even social expression. That means more weight. It's a vicious cycle. More calories, more weight, less self-esteem … more input, more calories … and the beat goes on.

This unfortunate cycle can only be broken in the mind. But it can be! Laurel Mellin, a dietician who teaches community medicine and pediatrics at the University of California at San Francisco School of Medicine, originally developed a simple 12-week program that proved so effective for overweight children, that it has been adopted for adults in more than 100 hospitals nationwide. In her book, *The Solution* (Regan

Books; 1st Harper edition June 1998), she argues that the key to real behavior modification that leads to effective weight loss is to focus on those same coping skills usually learned in childhood. For 18 years Mellin directed a well regarded child and adolescent program that is in use at over 400 hospitals across the nation and which has been shown to help heavy kids lose weight and keep it off.

The Solution borrows from different weight loss programs and then applies some common psychological techniques. For example, there is a hint of basic **cognitive therapy** which usually seeks to uncover and change one's self-defeating ways of thinking. Add to that the basics of Pavlov's **behavioral therapy** which simply reinforces good habits with rewards. To make it practical, the suggestion is to quietly pause five times a day to first ask two elementary questions: *'How am I feeling?'* and *'What do I really need?'* After identifying and labeling your true feelings in this way, you can find alternate ways to fulfil your needs by means other than eating. The next question then is: *'What can I do?'* The answers become insightful and empowering.

It seems simplistic, but some people who struggle with their weight are unable to accurately read and respond to their own emotions. They are prone to interpret all unnatural or disturbing feelings as hunger and try to satisfy them by eating, day and night.

However, eating is never the fundamental issue. Appetite is subject to normal feedback inhibition. When your body is starved, you get hungry and so you eat. But then, when your caloric and other nutritional needs are met, you are normally satisfied and even the sight or smell of food loses its sensual appeal. This is normal behavior. Extreme anorexics who avoid eating naturally, have a grossly distorted body image and consider their weight excessive even as they begin to wither away. Those prone to overeating and gluttony (bulimics being the extreme) have again emotional and psychological constraints that are truly pathological, but always secondary. Therefore, the focus must be, not so much on the act of eating per se, but on the *thought* of eating.

So it becomes clear that **thinking turns the key**.

How do you think of eating? How do you think of your body? How do you think of yourself? Now, ask those same questions again, but this time in reverse, and you'll always get the answers right. To discover yourself, apart from your body, is to win the emotional victory! That's true, and it's the only way to truly master your body and authenticate yourself.

Your true self can never be measured in pounds. Why? Because **Character is weightless. Identity is form-less. Worth is shape-less.** Your essential character, your true identity and your real worth are going to remain ... with or without a ten percent change in your weight. You may look better, you may feel better, you may even be much healthier, but the reality is that you will always remain you. There may be less of you or even more of you, but *you* will forever be *you*!

How liberating it is then, to fall in love with the essential you. It is so important to affirm that your self is your first responsibility. **That affirmation opens the door.** So, self control is the key. Thinking turns the key that opens the door to your weight control ... the door to your health ... the door to your future ... and the door to your new life. 'To be or not to be' has long been settled, but *'to be me, and only me'* - that is the challenge! To love and cherish the me that I am, despite the body that I have or wish I had - therein is success and victory!

To begin a weight loss program with an intrinsic sense of self is really the strongest asset that you can have. Your thinking turns the key of self-control and your affirmation of self-worth opens the door.

The Enzyme Diet™ Solution is an effective, proven method to lose weight and improve your health at the same time. But it is essentially your healthy mind and your intrinsic sense of worth that will make it work for you. A healthy mind is an indispensable precursor to a healthy body and a healthy weight.

The Amazing New Wonderful You!

Now that you have discovered your intrinsic self, it is appropriate to work on your total self. Every marketer knows the importance of packaging. The package that is *you* comes in a package that is *your body*. When that body becomes healthier, slimmer and more appealing, to yourself first and then to others too, your marketability in this interpersonal world will be markedly increased. That's also true. Everything about you can and probably will change.

You will have a new understanding of your weight problem and a handle on an effective, comprehensive solution - **The Enzyme Diet™ Solution**. You'll realize that this is more than just another diet. It is truly a solution. It defines a new perspective that sustains a new responsible lifestyle. You'll think differently and appreciate the value of feeding your cells and maintaining your metabolism, while losing your unwanted pounds. As you make your personal application, with such sensible and adequate nutrition, and a complementary exercise program, you will soon see the weight scales dropping and your health soaring. You will discover the exhilaration of a healthy and vibrant lifestyle that you will want to engage for a lifetime.

So you begin with cultivating a healthy mind and a clear, balanced mind-set. You appreciate who you are, but you also acknowledge what you could be in a slimmer, healthier body package. You take responsibility, you seize control and as you apply **The Enzyme Diet™ Solution,** you begin to experience a transformation.

Like the caterpillar that sheds its exoskeleton repeatedly until it learns to internalize its growth, rebuilding from the inside out - and only to emerge as a free and beautiful butterfly that can soar and travel for many miles - you too will experience a similar metamorphosis! You will shed unwanted pounds and begin to enjoy an amazing, new wonderful you. You will feel proud, liberated and powerful - all because you're in control. Your more healthy body will transport a more healthy mind and that mind will celebrate a renewed sense of self and worth. You will experience life as you know it could be and you will Celebrate!

Celebrate your Weight Loss! Celebrate your Wellness! Celebrate your Life!

CONGRATULATIONS!

$\mathscr{Appendix}$ 'A'

CAeDS®: The Science Behind It All
(If you really want to know)

This section is included as an Appendix only for those who have enough curiosity and would like a more in-depth discussion of the background science to CAeDS® and enzyme delivery in general.

1. THE ENZYMES OF CAeDS®

The use of enzymes to increase the nutritive value of food has long been established in the food industry. Over the last twenty five years, numerous studies have been conducted which show the advantage of using enzymes as pre-digestive factors to increase nutrient yields. While research on supplemental enzymes is limited, a large body of research has been created by the food processing and agricultural industries.

During the digestive process, the large naturally-occurring molecules in food are broken down by different classes of enzymes into smaller fragments for more easy absorption and assimilation.

· *Proteins* are split into small peptide fractions and constituent amino acids. This is engineered by the action of proteolytic enzymes known as **proteases and peptidases.**

· *Fats (lipids)* are broken into smaller free fatty acids and glycerol, mainly by the action of the enzymes known generally as **lipase.**

· *Carbohydrate (starch)* is degraded to simple sugars, mainly by the action of the enzymes known generally as **amylase.** *Disaccharides* are further broken down by **maltase** and **lactase** into simple sugars.

· *Cellulose and other fibers,* in contrast, are not efficiently digested and they provide the essential bulk to the diet for important functions in the gastro-intestinal tract. Some complex enzymes, like **cellulase** and **pectinase**, do effectively break down some plant cell walls and become important in the release of nutrients.

We'll discuss each of these four classes of digestive enzymes in turn to summarize briefly what we do know about them in terms of nutrient bioavailability.

Proteolytic Enzymes and Nutrient Bioavailability

Proteins in the diet are derived from both plant and animal sources. The structure of these proteins, especially around the linkage (or peptide bond) between the different amino acid building blocks, is different in these two sources of foods.

Plant-based foods can offer a unique problem for the digestive system of mammals, including man. The proteolytic enzymes of the mammalian gastrointestinal tract fail to completely digest certain plant proteins and usually leave a "core" polypeptide of about 20 to 30 amino acids [1]. In contrast, animal proteins are typically well digested in the mammalian digestive tract.

The plant protein "core" results from the fundamentally different make-up of some plant and animal proteins. The abundance of hydrophobic alkyl-groups in animal proteins is thought to lead to the enhanced digestion and hence, increased bioavailability of animal protein.

Most people consume a wide variety of protein sources but most nutritionists encourage the consumption of less meats and more vegetables, fruits, cereals and legumes. This is so, for a variety of very good reasons. That is good advice because of what these plant sources do *not* contain (e.g. high fat and cholesterol) as much as what they *do* contain (phytonutrients). Many studies have demonstrated the healthy benefits of predominantly vegetarian diets when engaged wisely.

Cereal grasses, algae, legumes and various other plants have been investigated as possible alternative protein sources. Historically, the protein content of these plants has been extracted via a combination of pressure and abrasion, both mechanical and chemical, in order to rupture the cells and release the nutritive contents. Unfortunately, this process releases only one third of the plant protein. Lignins and cellulosic *fibers trap the remaining protein* [2].

Increasingly, consumption of high fiber diets "has been associated with reductions in the digestibility and availability of protein, fats and other nutrients such as minerals, vitamins and carbohydrates" [3]. Yet high fiber diets are also the rage of many nutritionists since that tends to favor the health of the gastrointestinal tract in most significant ways. It reduces the risk of colon cancer and many other bowel diseases. That is probably the way to go, but note the price in reduced nutrient bioavailability and the obvious need for supplementary enzymes that is implicated with high fiber diets.

Investigation on the effects of proteolytic pre-digestion on a variety of seed proteins including sesame, peanut, chickpea and field bean, showed increased solubility and nutritive value [4]. Protease has been used to increase the nutritive value available from both alfalfa and clover (5).

What does all this mean in practical terms?

The complexity of structure and properties of proteins and peptides requires the combination of multiple protease enzymes to optimize digestion. Let us consider the reasons why. Proteins are made up of more than twenty different amino acids. Each unique combination presents a different three dimensional shape and so-called conformational characteristics (6). These give rise to different structure-property relationships. Each proteolytic enzyme has different bond specificities and thus, only **a combination of enzymes** would be expected to show the greatest rate of hydrolysis. Several issues are involved.

· **Bond specificity** is an ongoing area of research in enzymology. However, some work has been done on the various *Aspergillus* proteases. Peptidase enzymes break amino acids off the ends of the peptide chain. The peptidase of **The Enzyme Diet**™ possesses both amino-peptidase and carboxy-peptidase activities and thus is able to remove amino acids from *both ends* of the peptide chain.

To be more specific, the enzymes Protease FP26, Protease FP23, Protease FP610 and Bromelain, break at different points within the peptide chain, dependent upon their bond specificities. While these specificities have not been fully elucidated, significant differences in the action of these enzymes have been observed both in the laboratory and in digestive product usage.

· Another property of these enzymes is that their action is very dependent on **the acidity of their environment**. This is measured by a pH value, with low numbers corresponding to a more acid environment as found in the stomach, and higher values to a more alkaline environment such as in the intestines.

The pH optima and ranges of these enzymes are also an important benefit of combining these proteases. Protease FP26 has an optimal pH range of 2.0 to 6.0, Protease FP23 has an optimal pH range of 2.0 to 3.0, while Protease FP610 has an optimal pH range of 6.0 to 10.0 and Bromelain has an optimal pH range of 5.0 to 8.0. Together, these proteases provide proteolytic action **throughout the human digestive system**. That increases overall protein digestion and hence, bioavailability.

· Naturally occurring **enzyme inhibitors** are another consideration in supplementation of exogenous enzymes.

This can be illustrated by considering the main proteolytic enzymes pepsin and trypsin. Pepsin is the principal digestive enzyme of the stomach's (gastric) juice. It is formed from the precursor, pepsinogen, and hydrolyzes the peptide bond of proteins at low pH (high acid) values. Trypsin is more predominant in babies. It is formed in the small intestine from an inactive precursor provided by pancreatic secretions into the early part of the intestine (the duodenum). It is more active at the higher pH values of the intestine.

Various plant foods are known to possess potent trypsin inhibitors. Egg whites and soybeans are perhaps the best-known sources of trypsin inhibiting compounds. Perhaps that explains, in part, why egg whites are contra-indicated in young infants. These inhibitors are effective, due to the similarity of their structures to the binding site of trypsin. Supplementation of exogenous proteases with differing configurations of binding sites could therefore be, in principle, very beneficial.

Lipolytic Enzymes and Nutrient Bioavailability

Many people all over the world consume too much fat, usually animal fat. In some places, where a bowl of rice or corn is the staple diet, this is not an issue at all. Animal meats would sometimes be a luxury item there. But it is not uncommon, even in the developing world, to see individuals consuming high fat foods - cheap fast foods, low quality meats, dairy products and even some fish, for example. Fat impacts flavor, after cooking and frying (especially in oils), and tends to early satiety (feeling full). But high fat consumption is demanding.

As we keep repeating so you are sure not to miss the message, lipase enzymes digest fat, releasing free fatty acids and glycerol. Problems with fat digestion are believed to be prevalent among many modern consumers of popular high fat diets. These are particularly associated with highly processed, convenience and junk foods. Fat digestion is known to be a clinical problem with certain diseases, including pancreatitis and cystic fibrosis. Increased digestion of fats can increase the bioavailability of the fat-soluble nutrients like Vitamin E and Vitamin A.

Interestingly, research in the food industry has also shown that increasing fat hydrolysis can increase protein bioavailability from fish and other meats (7). Lipase has also been used to increase the nutritive value available from both alfalfa and clover (5).

Amylolytic Enzymes and Nutrient Bioavailability

Starch is abundant in the natural world where it serves as the primary energy source for plants, animals and humans. Starch consists of glucose polymers. These polymers exist in two basic compositions, amylose and amylopectin. Amylose, the minor constituent, consists of straight chains of glucose joined with alpha-1,4-glucosidic bonds. Amylopectin consists of branched glucose chains. The branching of the glucose chain occurs with the formation of an alpha-1,6-glucosidic bond. The ratio of amylose to amylopectin varies dependent upon the origin of the starch, but it is typically in the range of 1:3 to 1:4 (8).

Starch digestion is optimized with the **combination of the enzymes** alpha-amylase, glucoamylase and malt diastase. While alpha-amylase breaks glucose-glucose bonds at random points within the starch chain, malt diastase hydrolyzes the starch chain from the ends to create glucose dimers (maltose), and glucoamylase breaks single glucose molecules off the ends of the chain. The hydrolytic action of both alpha-amylase and malt diastase is blocked by the alpha-1,6-glucosidic bonds of amylopectin. The conformation of these limit dextrins prevents the active site of the enzymes from coming in contact with the glucose-glucose bonds, thus inhibiting hydrolysis. Glucoamylase hydrolyzes the alpha-1,6-glucosidic bond, freeing the chain for continued hydrolysis of the alpha-1,4-bonds (9).

Starches can sometimes **limit the absorption of proteins** and other important nutrients. Soybeans are a poor source of starch and the small amount available is tightly associated with the protein, actually interfering with the trypsin hydrolysis of the legume's protein. Supplementation of amylase removes this starch and frees the protein for proteolysis (10).

Just as for proteins, naturally occurring **enzyme inhibitors** are another consideration in considering supplementation of exogenous enzymes.

Various plant foods are known to possess potent alpha-amylase inhibitors. Grains, legumes and other seeds are the best known sources of these anti-enzyme compounds. Wheat albumin proteins contain a fraction that effectively inhibits human alpha-amylase but do not inhibit fungal amylase. Furthermore, it is established that significant anti-amylase activity survives processing and baking to interfere with normal digestion (1).

Fiber-breaking Enzymes and Nutrient Bioavailability

As mentioned above, the fiber content of plant foods can bind proteins and other nutrients. These nutrients are often entrapped within complex polysaccharide matrices - such matrices are often composed of lignins, cellulose, hemicellulose, pectins and other polysaccharides (11:8).

The fiber-breaking enzymes include cellulase, CereCalase™ and pectinase. Each of these enzymes consists of multiple enzymes that act on a number of different substrates. Together these enzymes help breakdown the case-like structure of the plant cell wall. This has major commercial applications.

The Fruit Juice Industry

In the juice industry, the plant cell wall limits the ability to extract juice. The cell wall must be broken open to improve extraction ratios. The historical methods of mechanical processing have several inherent problems including the production of heat. Heat can cause off-colors and bad flavor in the final product. Thus, the juice industry began researching enzymes as a means to break down the cell wall. The cell wall has been shown to be particularly troublesome with the extraction of orange juice, apple cider and pear cider. In the case of orange juice extraction, mechanical disruption of the sacs is somewhat random. Many juice sacs are missed completely.

With the addition of enzymes under the right conditions (time and temperature), all juice sacs are readily broken open. In the orange juice industry, combinations of cellulase, hemicellulase (CereCalase™) and pectinase are used to disrupt the cell walls. This potent combination essentially liquefies the cell wall. Juice extraction can be increased up to 95% with the use of enzymes.

Therefore, enzymes have become the primary method of processing in the juice industry (12). It is more efficient.

Emphasis should be placed on the fact that the goal of CAeDS® is not to liquefy the fibers that humans consume as part of a healthy diet. The physical bulk provided by the fiber is necessary to maintain healthy bowel habits. In addition, modern research has discovered many benefits with fiber consumption including cholesterol-lowering effects and decreased incidence of various types of cancer.

In a CAeDS®-delivered product like The Enzyme Diet™, the goal is to improve the bioavailability of nutrients by disrupting the fiber matrix. CAeDS® can effectively destroy the cell wall, which opens up the cell and releases nutrients and bioactives so that they are available for absorption.

Another interesting fact worth noting from the juice industry is the effect of enzymes on the level of color and aroma components. Industry research indicates that enzyme usage increases the amount of color and aroma agents. These findings are especially interesting when anthocyanidins are considered.

Research in the grape juice and wine industries shows that enzyme usage increases the level of anthocyanidins in the final product (13;14). Anthocyanidins are antioxidant compounds that are the active ingredients of hawthorn, grape seed extract, gingko and bilberry. All of these items have very similar chemical structures.

If the juice industry by using enzymes can increase the level of these chemicals in their juice products, then CAeDS® blends should increase the bioavailability of such antioxidants in dietary supplements.

The Agricultural Industry

Just as fiber is a problem in the juice industry, it is also a problem for animals trying to digest their food. Certain nutrients are very readily bound to fibers and thus are unavailable to the animals. Research over the last 30 years shows conclusively that enzyme supplementation of cereal based diets, especially rye and barley, is highly beneficial to the growth of animals.

Another area of research is the improvement of protein utilization from vegetable sources including soy, peas and oilseeds (15).

The agricultural industry is a master of recycling. The industry often takes inexpensive waste products from other industries and explores the nutritional value for livestock. Expenses must be kept to a minimum, so the agricultural industry continues to develop processing methods to improve utilization of these industrial wastes.

As a result, the agricultural industry has invested significant research into trying to make cottonseed, grape seed and various other substances suitable for livestock consumption. The results have been favorable, with many enzyme-modified "wastes" becoming suitable feedstuffs.

In the agricultural market, the most important part of raising animals is for each animal to become fat and healthy. If the animal does not get enough utilizable fats, sugars and proteins, the animal is not going to be healthy and the farmer loses money.

Cell wall structure varies with each plant. Different sugars are present at different levels dependent upon the particular species. Therefore, optimization of the feedstuffs requires supplementation of *different enzymes*.

Research by the agricultural industry has broken major feedstuffs into four groups based upon the structure of the cell wall. Corn and sorghum have been identified as the ideal diet, with livestock growing and getting fat quickly. Cost analysis of enzyme supplementation with this group of feedstuffs shows that any slight improvement does not merit the additional cost.

This is not the case with the other three groups where enzyme supplementation has been shown to be quite beneficial and well worth the added cost. Beta-glucanases (CereCalase™) and pectinases have been shown to be the most beneficial enzymes.

Specific Examples of Agricultural Research
· Treatment of alfalfa with a combination of cellulase and pectinase was found **to enhance protein availability** from the leaves by nearly 50% (16). Cellulase was used to increase digestibility of the protein in wheat bran by 35% and rats fed bran with cellulase grew 25% faster than control rats (17). Studies using *Aspergillus niger* cellulase for predigestion consistently show significantly increased nutritive value of vegetable foodstuffs.

· The use of polysaccharidases, such as cellulase, can **increase the calories per unit weight** of plant foods by transforming a portion of the fiber into utilizable sugars. In this way, plant foods that are low in carbohydrates can be modified to improve their total nutritional value.

· The use of cellulase and hemicellulase **to digest the cell walls of vegetable feeds for increased digestibility** is widely accepted in the animal feed industry - particularly for cattle, pigs and poultry.

· An enzyme complex isolated from *Trichoderma viride* including cellulase and other fiber digesting enzymes was fed to mature hens and was **shown to increase energy and nutrient utilization** (18). Research on the use of various enzyme preparations has been conducted for over 30 years and clearly establishes that the digestibility of nutrients and productivity of animals can be increased (19) (20).

· Glucanases have been used **to increase the protein availability** in soybeans from 75% to 95% (21). A proposed mechanism for beta-glucanase is that it functions to decrease viscosity caused by beta-glucan gums in the digestive tract. Soy meal is pre-digested with pectinolytic enzymes, cellulase and hemicellulase, to increase the availability of soluble carbohydrates and utilizable sugars, thus improving the nutritional content of the legume (22).

· Additionally, alpha-galactosidase supplementation has been shown to benefit the animal industry. Many feedstuffs contain the same substances, raffinose-series sugars that cause gastrointestinal discomfort in humans upon the consumption of beans and cruciferous vegetables. Animals (and humans) have microorganisms that ferment, (or eat), the raffinose-series sugars, producing some absorbable sugars and gas. The animal gains some benefits from this **microbial fermentation**, which releases an average of 50 to 60% of the potential from the galactosaccharides. Yet, when raising livestock this 50 to 60% is not enough if there is an inexpensive way of increasing that level of potential energy. When each pound the animal gains equals money in a rancher's pocket, enzyme supplementation becomes a very practical solution.

· Another enzyme of interest to the agricultural industry is phytase (as in CereCalase™). Phytic acid binds organic phosphorus with inositol. In vegetables, phytic acid tends to bind minerals including calcium and zinc, making them inaccessible to absorption. One of the advantages of phytase is that it breaks down phytate, releasing the phosphorus and other minerals to become bioavailable (23) (24). On the average, less than 50% of the phosphorus of any given cereal is available to the animal. Supplementation of phytase can **increase that level of phosphorus as well as other bound minerals**. Another advantage of using this enzyme in the agricultural industry is the reduction of phosphate-containing waste, which is a serious pollutant of the environment (25).

The fact that these enzymes can also offer direct benefit for human beings is also an area of increasing research. Recently, several groups of scientists have begun exploring the role of certain enzymes in improving health and nutrition (26). Most notable among this research are **the effects of phytase on improving mineral absorption in humans.**

Phytic acid is a mineral-binding agent that reduces the bioavailability of certain minerals such as zinc, iron, magnesium and calcium (27). This mineral-binding substance is prevalent in many plant foods including cereal grains and legumes. For this reason, it is often advantageous to break down the phytic acid-mineral complex. Research by Ann-Sofie Sanderg indicates that dietary phytase is critical for human digestion of phytate. This research (26) has also noted that supplemental phytase from *Aspergillus niger* increases iron absorption in humans.

2. THE MINERAL ACTIVATORS OF CAeDS®

Minerals perform a wide variety of essential functions in the human body. Iron in red blood cell hemoglobin is critical for vital oxygen transport via the circulation. Certain minerals (sodium, potassium) are involved in the regulation of fluid and electrolyte balance. Others (especially calcium) provide skeletal rigidity, and some are needed for proper nerve and muscle performance. One of the most important roles of minerals is their key role in metabolism. Minerals are required components in the metabolic enzyme systems. These metabolic enzyme systems are responsible for the breakdown of carbohydrates and fats to release energy, and the creation of new proteins for many indispensable life functions. In addition, vitamins, hormones, peptides, and other substances require minerals to help regulate the body's metabolic systems. If the body is lacking in key minerals required for these enzymes and hormones to function, metabolism may slow.

The fact that enzymes require cofactors in order to function properly is well established and can be found in most physiology and biochemistry textbooks. For example,

> *"Many enzymes are completely inactive when they are isolated in a pure state. Evidently some of the ions and smaller organic molecules that were removed in the purification procedure are needed for enzyme activity. These ions and smaller organic molecules are called co-factors and co-enzymes."* (28)

These co-factors are most often minerals, such as calcium, magnesium, zinc, copper, chromium and others. Each enzyme requires different minerals to be optimally activated. In the absence of the co-factor some enzymes do not have a properly shaped active site and may not function at all (28).

Recognizing the need for enzymes to promote proper digestion and that these essential enzymes are possibly mineral activated and certainly dependent upon specific minerals, members of the Infinity2 Formulation Team theorized that supplementing with specific minerals would increase enzymatic activity.

But not all minerals are created equal. Just because a supplement contains a specific milligram amount of a mineral, such as zinc or calcium, doesn't mean that the mineral is in a form that the body can readily absorb and use. As with any nutrient, whether it be protein, fats, carbohydrates, or vitamins, simply ingesting minerals is not enough. The nutrients must be readily absorbable, or, in other words "bioavailable." Otherwise, they are nothing more than waste material in the body.

To provide support for this theory, research studies were conducted demonstrating that supplementation with amino acid chelated minerals increased disaccharidase enzyme activity at the intestinal membrane. The details of these studies can be found in the **Albion Patent US #5,882,685** (29).

Only bioavailable minerals enter and enhance the body's metabolic processes and contribute to the maintenance and production of healthy tissues.

Inorganic mineral salts (i.e. chloride, sulfate, carbonate, ascorbate) have low bioavailability because they are poorly absorbed and have poor retention. The estimated absorption rates for mineral salts range from only 5% to 40% depending on the mineral, the pH of the intestine and the interaction with other nutrients in the intestinal lumen (30;31). Unfortunately, such inorganic salt forms of minerals, are the most commonly used in the food and supplementation industries.

Minerals that are true amino acid chelates, however, are much more bioavailable. The **absorption rates are three to six times greater** than mineral salts and have twice the retention (32-35)

In addition to the research and patents demonstrating the effectiveness of mineral chelates in enhancing enzyme activity, research has demonstrated that **these mineral chelates are delivered on a cellular level** (36) as was patented in the **Albion Patent US #4,863,898.**

The mineral chelates used in **The Enzyme Diet**™ have been put through an exhaustive array of scientific tests to verify that they are true chelates. Many studies have consistently shown that these mineral chelates are:

- **Highest in tolerence**
- **Lowest in toxicity**
- **Highest in bioavailability**
- **100% in nutrient density**
- **Superior in physiological activity**

Many companies claim to produce chelates, but in truth, research has disclosed that these so called "Cheap Chelates" are really salts, or complexes (minerals wet-blended with hydrolyzed protein). They are not true chelates. **The formation of a nutritionally functional chelate is a lot more sophisticated and expensive than simply mixing minerals and protein together.** That is why in **The Enzyme Diet™** only Albion's patented chelates are used. In fact, Albion has earned over **50 patents** related to mineral chelates. These patents guarantee that no one else can produce a nutritionally functional chelate that compares to Albion's mineral chelates.

Most low calorie diets are low in key minerals and other nutrients required for metabolism. As a result, individuals lose weight at the expense of a reduced metabolism. Supplying optimal amounts of vitamins and minerals to support metabolism during weight loss may prevent the reduction in metabolism that often occurs with low calorie diets. Supporting the body's metabolic enzymes is a key premise behind the formulation of **The Enzyme Diet™**. It provides enzymes and patented amino acid chelated minerals to support the body's metabolism during weight loss. These patented minerals are absorbed and utilized by the body more effectively than any other forms of minerals and help ensure that the minerals reach the cells where metabolism occurs.

3. EVIDENCE FOR CAeDS® AT WORK

What's the evidence that CAeDS® is more than just a bright idea? Does it really work? Perhaps the best demonstration of the value of a tissue delivery system was presented by Dr. Ashmead for studies with the enzyme SuperOxide Dismutase. Let's review that.

The production of free radicals in the body is an essential consequence of the normal biochemical and physiological processes. But generally they are kept under control by the primary antioxidants, the cytoprotective enzymes and the secondary antioxidants such as the transition metal and heme protein binders, and the interceptors of propagating radical reactions. The oxidative stress from free radical production occurs when the balance between these oxidants and the antioxidants is tripped in favor of the free radicals. This could be from exogenous agents of oxidative stress, radiation, trauma, drug activation, oxygen excess or endogenous oxidative stress associated with many pathological states. Specifically, free radicals target the polyunsaturated fats that compose the lipid portion of cell membranes leading to peroxidation, cellular damage and eventually disease.

Not much can be done about the ultra fast hydroxyl, alkoxyl or alkyl-dioxyl radicals. On the other hand, the less reactive hydrogen peroxide and superoxides can be disposed of by interception with superoxide dismutase (SOD). There are two known forms of SOD found in mammalian tissues. One is a copper/zinc (Cu/Zn) containing enzyme present in the cytoplasm of most cells, and the other is a manganese (Mn) containing enzyme found in the mitochondria. Both enzymes catalyse the same reaction and are specific to this sub-

strate only. There needs to be a continuing dietary supply of these three minerals in order for the SOD enzyme to function.

Studies using the jejunal segments of rat intestines have clearly demonstrated that when either of these minerals was chelated to amino acids, there was
greater intestinal absorption in vitro than from the standard 'cheap' metal salts.
(37) Further, the important question then arises: *After absorption, are those
chelates deposited in the tissues in greater quantities, or are they simply excreted into the urinary systems or returned to the lower bowel without being metab-
olized?* In vivo radioisotope studies help provide the answers to these questions.

Table 15			
Mean 65Zn* in Tissues			
Tissues	65Zn Amino Acid Chelate	65ZnCl2	% Increase
Muscle	186	153	22
Heart	1,457	1,433	2
Liver	10,250	7,529	36
Kidney	8,629	7,797	11
Brain	541	444	22
*Corrected counts/minute/gm of wet tissue			

Table 16			
Mean 54Mn* in Tissues			
	54Mn Amino	54MnCl2	% Increase
Heart	107	36	197
Liver	106	52	104
Kidney	97	80	21
Spleen	397	190	109
Lung	56	54	4
Small Intestine	141	89	58
Muscle	28	22	27
Bone	266	112	138
*Corrected counts/minute/gm of wet tissue			

The rates of deposition in different tissues in *live rats* was monitored
with radioactive isotopes to demonstrate that the chelates were deposited in the
different tissues in greater quantities than with the inorganic salts. **Tables 15**
and **16** summarize this increase (38).

The bigger question then becomes: *Once deposited in the tissues, are
the minerals metabolically active or do they simply reside there?* In vivo studies using beef cattle demonstrated increased erythrocyte SOD activity in the animals supplemented with the amino acid chelates compared to the inorganic salts.
In another study involving 24 healthy, non smoking females of average age 23.9

years, the effect of manganese amino acid chelate supplementation on their lymphocyte MnSOD activity was measured compared to placebo over four months. The results illustrated in **Figure 3** showed that the increase in MnSOD activity was significant (P<0.01) (39).

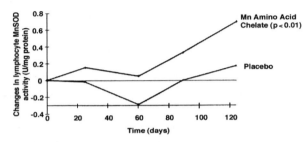

Figure 3   Changes in lymphocyte MnSOD activity over time in 24 women supplemented with Manganese Amino Acid Chelate or placebo.

At a conference on antioxidants and disease prevention held in London, England, in 1989, Professor Anthony T. Diplock stated that free radicals are probably involved in a number of diseases. The prevention of these diseases involves dioxygen reduction to water through the involvement of several active intermediates.

> *"The control of this depends on the integrity of the enzyme system that requires adequate intake of ... copper, zinc and manganese; if their level of intake is low, proliferation of active oxygen metabolites may occur. Targets for attacks are DNA, proteins and polyunsaturated phospholipids. Peroxidation of polyunsaturated phospholipids will result in disruption of membrane architecture."*

The data above demonstrate that when these essential antioxidant mineral nutrients are ingested in the form of amino acid chelates, the total requirement for these minerals was reduced due to their greater bioavailability. Furthermore, Cu/Zn SOD and Mn SOD activity increased, presumably as a result of the chelates' greater metabolic activity after absorption. From a free radical perspective, these three antioxidant minerals, when in the amino acid chelate form, become of primary value biologically by increasing SOD activity, which in turn may restrict the damage that reactive free radicals can produce in the cells and tissues of our bodies.

Let's go a step further. Most rheumatoid arthritis patients have increased copper requirements as a consequence of their inflammation. Most do not consume adequate dietary copper to maintain proper SOD activity in their bodies. However, a study from Purdue University on 23 rheumatoid arthritis patients compared to 48 healthy age - matched controls showed that the Cu/Zn SOD activity is increased significantly (P < 0.001) after four weeks of supplementation with the copper amino acid chelates. **(Table 17)** (40). The use of amino acid chelates to enhance the immune system in general was described by Dr. R.T. Coffee in Dr. Ashmead's classic review Monograph.

Table 17		
Cu/Zn SOD Activity Changes in Erythrocytes of in Rheumatoid Arthritics and Healthy Controls		
	Presupplementation	Postsupplementation
Controls (48)	3368 ± 364	$3486\pm443b$
Arthritics (23)	2934 ± 456^a	$3448\pm446c$

* Units/ml packed cells

a   P<0.001 Significant difference from controls
b   P<0.005 Significant difference from presupplementation
c   Significant increase from presupplemented arthritics (P<0.001)

To demonstrate *in vitro* the effects of the CAeDS® system of botanical constituent delivery, Infinity2's *St. John's Wort* formula was subjected to incubation in a simulated gastric environment and sampled at various intervals. Chromatographic analysis was then applied to determine what changes were taking place. There are two known actions or mechanisms at work in these systems:

  i. An overall increase in the "release" or "solubility" of herbal components from their plant matrix.
 ii. An herbal constituent itself may be enzymatically hydrolyzed.

Over time, a fairly dramatic enzyme-hydrolysis of rutin into quercetin was observed. Other effects, though not as dramatic, included an overall increase in both chlorogenic acid and caffeic acid.

Although the analysis was limited by availability of commercial standards, complexities of herbal constituents, etc., definite enzymatic effects were demonstrated. They serve well to indicate the potential synergistic relationships possible with CAeDS®.

Appendix '**B**'

Delightful Flavorful Recipes*

The preparation of **The Enzyme Diet**™ typically calls for you to first add 2 level scoops of the fine powder (in natual French Vanilla or Cocoa flavors) to 8 fluid oz. or 1 cup of cold water or skim milk. You then use a blender or shaker to mix it well and drink the original meal replacement shake immediately.

But you can become creative and satisfy your taste buds with a variety of other flavors that can easily be made by using your same shaker or blender, and adding some tasteful goodies to your French Vanilla base.

Here are some suggestions, **courtesy of Susan B. Tucker**:

- Take 8 oz water or skim milk
     or 4 oz 'fresh squeezed' orange juice plus 4 oz water
     or 4 oz water plus 1/2 cup of crushed ice

- Add 2 scoops of The Enzyme Diet, then

- Add *one* of the following:

     - 1/2 teaspoon cinnamon, nutmeg, ginger or favorite spice
     - 1/2 banana (2.5 oz)
     - 1/4 cup berries
     - 1/2 cup fresh pineapple (or crushed), no sugar added
     - 2 cups melon or cantaloupe
     - 1/2 peach (peeled and pitted)
     - 1/2 papaya
     - 1/2 mango

- Blend until smooth.

However, remember that adding additional fruits or flavorings will change the calorie and or fat intake per serving. When using fruits, make sure that the fruit is unsweetened and without additives. You can easily change the consistency of the shake by diluting with a small amount of water to your satisfaction. **Now Enjoy!**

* *For more detailed information on the recipes, see www.infinity2.com*

Appendix 'C'

Workout Exercises

Here are some simple routines that you can do at home. Begin slowly and gradually increase the number of repetitions to fill your 30 minute workout.

- *Standing Squat:*

    Stand upright with your feet shoulder-width apart, toes pointing forward or slightly outward. Keeping the back straight and bending the knees, squat down in seven seconds, until the thigh is parallel to the floor. Make sure that you stay flat-footed and ensure that the knees do not go over the toes as you squat down. Go back to an upright position, utilizing a seven-second count. Do not lock the knees out at the top, immediately start the downward motion, again using a seven-second count. Perform this exercise to failure or 15 repetitions.

- *Duck Squat:*

    Stand upright, with the heels approximately 24 inches apart and the toes pointing outward. Place a two-by-six inch board or thick phone book under the heels to elevate them. Keeping the back straight and bending the knees, squat down in seven seconds until the thighs are parallel to the floor, and then, taking seven seconds, slowly return to a standing position. Again, be sure that the knees do not go over the toes. Do not lock your knees out at the top, but immediately start the downward motion again. Remember to breathe constantly throughout the exercise.

- *Lunges:*

    Standing at one end of a room, step forward with one foot, using a slightly longer than normal step. Allow the knee of the trailing leg to lower until the knee almost touches the floor, without the front knee going out over the front toe. Stand up slightly, and bring the trailing leg forward slowly, taking another step without resting in the middle; again allow the back leg to lower until the knee almost touches the floor. Continue this lunging motion across the room, and then turn around and go back. This movement does not use the Super-Slow count but should be done slowly and smoothly. Maintain good posture, making sure the head and shoulders are upright.

    For those with arthritis or other joint problems, you can do the mini-lunge instead. To perform a mini lunge, step forward with one foot, using a slightly longer than normal step. Bend both knees and slowly lower your body toward the floor, but only go partially down. Be sure that the front knee does not go over your toes. Then slowly straighten both legs to stand up. Rather than stepping forward, continue to slowly raise and lower in one place for 15 repetitions. Then switch and place the opposite leg forward. Repeat 15 repetitions.

- *Standing Calf Rises:*

Place the balls of the feet on the edge of a two-by-six inch board or on the edge of a step, with the heels hanging off the edge. Lock the knees, and balance the body by holding onto a chair or stair rail. Gradually raise the heels to a count of seven seconds until you are standing on your tiptoes. Be sure to extend up as high as possible. Lower the heels in seven seconds, until a deep stretch is achieved.

- *Kneeling Leg Lift:*

Place knees and hands on the floor, keeping the back straight so shoulders are parallel to the hips. Using seven seconds to complete the motion, keeping the knee bent at a right angle, extend one leg back and up, until the thigh is parallel to the floor. Squeeze and flex the leg and buttocks at the top of the motion. Perform the same motion with the other leg, continuing to perform the upward motion in seven seconds and the downward in seven. Do as many as possible, up to 15 on each leg.

- *Push-up:*

With this exercise, there are several ways to start easily and then progress. Most people should start this exercise using a negative-only technique. Assume a standard push-up position on the toes with hands and body stiff. The hands should be placed slightly wider than shoulder-width. Lower the body to the floor by slowly bending the arms to a count of seven seconds. Do not try to push yourself up into the top position. When you reach the floor, bend the knees, straighten the arms and get back onto the toes and stiffen the body once again. Begin another repetition, lowering yourself in seven seconds.

Beginners may begin doing half push ups with knees on the floor. Slowly advance to full push ups as you get stronger.

- *Door Row:*

Roll up a towel and grab it with your hands near the middle of the towel, about six inches apart. Facing the narrow edge of an open door, place the middle of the towel against the door's edge just above the door knobs. Loop the ends of the towel around the knobs on each side. Slide the hands down to the end of the towel, and place the feet on either side of the door. Lean the torso down and back, and bend at the knees so thighs are parallel with the floor and the arms are extended. Stay in this position, keeping your torso angled away from the door. Keeping the elbows in, and using a 7-second count, pull yourself up until the chest meets the hands. Flex the back muscles. Lower yourself back down in seven seconds. You can control the amount of resistance by altering the angle of your torso. Do as many as possible, maintaining good form, up to 15.

- *Lat Pull Down:*

     You will need a towel and a partner. Sit backward on a chair, with the hands high above the head, holding the ends of the rolled-up towel. Have your partner hold the middle of the towel. While your partner provides continuous resistance by pulling up, pull the towel down behind your head in a slow smooth motion (seven-second count). Have your partner then reverse the resistance by pulling down while you push the towel back up to the starting position, again in seven seconds. Continue to fatigue or to 15 repetitions.

- *Tricep Extension:*

     For the Seated Tricep Extension, you will need two chairs. Start with the heels on one chair and place the other chair far enough away so that the palms of the hands are on the edge of the chair just behind the body, slightly more than shoulder-width apart. Keep the body upright. There should be a parallel line between the heels, the hips and the palms of hands. Lower the body in seven seconds until the shoulders are parallel with the elbows, then raise the body back up in seven seconds. At the top of the motion, squeeze the triceps and then immediately begin to lower using the seven-second count.

- *Arm Curl:*

     Stand erect with a weight in each hand. Hold the elbows close to the sides, never allowing the arms to move behind the body. Bending at the elbow, curl the weights up to the shoulders in seven seconds; then, lower again in seven seconds. It is important to maintain good posture and not swing the arms from side to side or to arch the back while performing this exercise. When you can do 15 repetitions increase the resistance by adding more weight or working with a partner as described below.

- *Lateral Raise:*

     Stand erect with the arms at your sides and a weight in each hand. Keeping the arms straight with the wrists slightly curled under, raise weights to just above shoulder height in seven seconds. Pause, then lower smoothly in seven seconds. Household items can be used for weights, such as soup cans or gallon cartons filled with different amounts of water to vary resistance. Increase the weight when you are able to do 15 slow repetitions in good form.

- *Crunches:*

Lie face up on the floor with the hands on the stomach. Bring the heels to within two feet of the buttocks and raise the toes off the ground. From this position, lift the shoulders and back off the floor as high as possible keeping the chin up and the neck straight. Try to hold the highest position for seven seconds. You will notice that only about a third of a standard sit-up is being performed. Lower the shoulders and back to the floor in seven seconds. Continue, doing as many crunches as possible. Unlike other exercises, crunches may be done daily.

ல References ல

Chapter 1

1. *US Surgeon General's Call to Action to Prevent and Decrease Overweight and Obesity*, US Dept of Health and Human Services, Centers for Disease Control and Prevention (CDC), December 13, 2001.
2. Centers for Disease Control and Prevention, *Morbidity and Mortality Weekly Report*, Sep 7, 2001.
3. US Dept of Health and Human Resources. Physical Activity and Health: A Report of the Surgeon General, CDC, 1996.
4. Clinical Guidelines in the Identification, Evaluation and Treatment of Overweight and Obesity in Adults, NIH, National Heart, Lung and Blood Institute, June 1998. *Obes Res.*, 1998; 6 (2): 97-106.

Chapter 2

1. *Commercial Weight Loss Products and Programs. What Consumers Stand to Gain and Lose*, A Public Conference, Oct. 16-17, 1997, Washington, DC.
2. Willett WC, Dietary Fat and Obesity: an unconvincing relation. *Am J Clin Nutr* 1998; 68, 1149-50
3. Westman, Eric, Presented at the Annual Scientific Meeting of the American Heart Association, November, 2002
4. Pittler MH et al. Randomized, double-blind trials of chitosan for body weight reduction. *Eur J Clin Nutr* 1999, 53, 379-381.
5. Anderson, James W. et al, Longterm weight-loss maintenance, a meta-analysis of US studies. *Am J Clin Nutr* 2001, 74: 579-584.
6. Heber D., Ashley JM, Wang EJ, Elashoff RM. Clinical Evaluation of a minimal intervention meal replacement regimen for weight reduction. *Jour Amer Coll of Nutr* 1994, 6, 608-614.
7. Ditschuneit HH, Flechtner-Mors M, Adler G. The effectiveness of meal replacement with diet shakes on long term weight loss and weight maintenance (abstract). Eighth International Congress on Obesity, Paris, 1998.
8. 'O' The Oprah Magazine, January, 2003, pg 53-56.

Chapter 3

1. Leibel RL. Is Obesity due to a heritable difference in 'set point' for adiposity? *West J Med* 1990: 153: 429-431.
2. Leibel RC, Rosenbaum M and Hirsch J. Changes in Energy Expenditure

Resulting from Altered Body Weight. *New England Journal of Medicine* 1995: 332, 621-628.
3. Weinsier Rl and Fried SK, *Amer J Clin Nutr 2000, 72 (5): 1088-1094*

Chapter 4

1. Grossman M.I. et al., "The effect of dietary composition on pancreatic enzymes," *Amer Jour Physiol.* 1943, 140:676-682.
2. Grossman M I et al., "On the mechanism of the adaptation of pancreatic enzymes to dietary composition," *Amer Jour Physiol.* 1944, 141: 38-41.
3. Ambrus J L, Lassman H B, DeMarchi J J, "Absoprtion of exogenous and endogenous proteolytic enzymes." *Clin. Pharmacol. Ther.* 1967, 8, 362-368.
4. Phelan J J et al., *Clin. Sci. Molec. Med.* (1977) 53, 35-43
5. McCarthy C E, *Proc. Nutr. Sci.* (1976) 35, 37-40
6. *Absorption of Orally Administered Enzymes* (Springer-Varlag, 1995), printed in Germany and edited by Prof. MLG Gardner (Univ. of Bradford, UK) and K.-J. Steffens (Rheinische Friedrick - Wilhelms - Universitat, Germany).

Chapter 6

1. Underwood, Anne, "The Great Nutrition Debate," *Newsweek*, March 6, 2000.

Chapter 8

1.   Foster - Powell K., Miller J B ., International Tables of Glycemic Index, *Am. J. Clin. Nutr.,* 1995, 62: 8715-8935.
2. Somersall, A C and Bounous, G., *Breakthrough in Cell Defense*, (GOLDENeight Publishers, 1998)

Chapter 9

1. Heber, David, *The Resolution Diet* (Avery, 1999) p. 135
2. *Physical Activity and Health: A Report of the Surgeon General*, Atlanta, GA., US Dept. of Health and Human Services, Centers for Disease Control and Prevention, National Center for Chronic Disease Prevention and Health Promotion, 1996.
3. The Center for Disease Control, "Progress toward achieving the 1990 national objectives for physical fitness and exercise." *MMWR* 1989; 38: 449-453.
4. Blair, S. "Physical fitness and all causes of mortality. A prospective study of healthy men and women." *JAMA*, 1989, 262: 2395-2401.
5. Westcott, Wayne: Strength fitness: *Physiological Principles and Training Techniques* (WC Brown Publishers, Dubuque, IA., 1989, p. xiii)

6. Fallon, Sally and Mary G. Enig, "Diet and Heart Disease: Not what you think," *Consumers Research*, July 1996, p.19.
7. Gutman R. A. et al., Long term hypertriglyceridemia and glucose intolerance in rats fed chronically an isocaloric sucrose-rich diet, *Metab. Clin. Exp.*, 1987, 36: 1013-1020.
8. Anderson R.A. and Kozlovsky A.J., Am. J. *Clin. Nutri.*, 1985; 41, 1177-1183.
9. Davis C.M. and Vincent J.B., Chromium in carbohydrate and lipid metabolism, *J. Biol. Inorg. Chem.*, 1997, 2, 675-679.
10. Stearns D.M. et al, Chromuim (III) p icolinate produces chromosome damage in Chinese hamster ovary cells, *FASEB J.*, 1995, 9, 1643-1648.

Chapter 10

1. Shaklee, Forrest C., *Reflections on a Philosophy* (Benjamin Co., 1973), p.26
2. Hill, Napoleon, *Think and Grow Rich* (Ballentine Publishing Group, May 1976)

Appendix A

1. Schwimmer, S. *Source Book of Food Enzymology.* Westport, CT, AVI Publishing Company Inc. 1981, 621-629.
2. Borgstrom, G. *Principles of Food Science: Food microbiology and Biochemistry.* New York, the McMillan Company. 1968, 433.
3. Schneeman, B. O. and D. Gallaher. Effects of dietary fiber on digestive enzyme activity and bile acids in the small intestine. *Proc. Soc. Exp. Biol. Med.* 180: 409-414, 1985.
4. Sreekantiah, K. R., H. Ebine, T. Ohta, and M. Nakano. Enzyme processing of vegetable protein foods. *Food Tech* 23: 1055-1061, 1969.
5. Edwards, G.W. and Edwards, A. W. *Alfalfa extracts.* (3,833,738). 9-10-1974. Ref Type: Patent
6. Fox, S. I. *Human Physiology.* Dubuque, Iowa, Wm. C. Brown Publishers. 1993.
7. Burkholder, L., P. R. Burkholder, A. Chu, N. Kostyk, and O. A. Roels. Fish fermentation. *Food Tech* 22: 1278-1284, 1968.
8. Salisbury, F. B. and C. W. Ross. *Plant Physiology.* Belmont, CA, Wadsworth Publishing Company. 1985.
9. *Modern Nutrition in Health and Disease.* Baltimore, Williams and Wilkins. 1994.
10. Boonvisut, S. and J. R. Whitaker. Effect of heat, amylase and disulfide bond cleavage on the in vitro digestibility of soybean proteins. *J Agric Food Chem* 24:1130-1135, 1976.
11. Halberg, L., L. rossander, and A. B. Skanberg. Phytates and the inhibitory

effect of bran on iron absorption in man. *Am. J. Clin. Nutr* 45: 988-996, 1987.

12 Madden, D. R. The use of enzymes in the manufacture of fruit juices. Practical Biotechnology. 1995 Ref Type: Electronic Citation

13. Gump, B. H. and Halght, K. G. A preliminary study of industrial enzyme preparations for color extraction/stability in red wines. Viticulture and Encology Research Center. 1995. Ref Type: Electronic Citation

14. Ough, C. S., A. C. Noble, and D. Temple. Pectic enzyme effects on red grapes. *Am. J. Enol. Vitic.* 26: 195-200, 1975.

15. Saint-Rat, L. Enzymatic extraction of proteins from various oilseed cakes. *C. R. Seances Acad. Agric.* 57: 826-830, 1971.

16. Mudgett, R. E., R. Rufner, R. Bahracharya, K. Kim, and K. Rajagopalan. Enzymatic effects on cell rupture in plant protein recovery. *J. Food Biochem* 2: 185-207, 1978.

17. 29. Saunders, R. M. and G. O. Kohler. Enzymatic processing of wheat bran. *Cereal Chem.* 49: 436-443, 1972.

18. Vranges, V. and C. Wrenk. Influence of Trichoderma viride enzyme complex on nutrient utilization and performance of laying hens in diets with and without antibiotic supplementation. *Poult. Sc.* 75: 551-555, 1996.

19. Modyanov, A. V. and V. R. Zel'ner. Application of Enzyme Supplements. In Rechcigl, M., Jr., ed. *CRC Handbook of Nutrititional Supplements*, Volume II, Agric. Use. Boca Raton, FL, CRC Press. 1983, 133-146.

20. Cowan, W. D. Animal Feed. In Godfrey, T. and S. West, eds. *Industrial Enzymology*. New York, Stockton Press. 1996.

21. Abdo, K.M. and A. King. Enzymatic modificatio of the extractability of protein from soybeans, Glycine max. *J Agric Food Chem* 15: 83-87, 1967.

22. Uhlig, H. and Grampp, E. *Soya meal treatment* (3,640,723). 2-8-1972. Ref. Type: Patent

23. Sebastian, S., S. P. Touchburn, E. R. Chavez, and P. C. Lague. The effects of supplemental microbial phytase on the performance and utilization of dietary calcium, phosphorus, copper, and zinc in broiler chickens fed corn-soybean diets *Poult. Sci.* 75: 729-736, 1996.

24. Murray, A. C., R. D. Lewis, and H. E. Amos. The effect of microbial phytase in perl millet-soybean meal diet on apparent digetibility and retentio of nutrients, serum mineral concentration, and bone mineral density of nursery pigs. *J. Animal. Sci.* 75: 1284-1291, 1997.

25. Sohail, S. S. and D. A. Roland. Fabulous Phytase: Phytase proving helpful to poultry producers and environment. Highlights of *Ag. Res.* 46: 1999.

26. Sandberg, A. S., L. Rossander-Hulthen, and M. Turk. Dietary Aspergillus niger phytase increases iron absorption in humans. *J. Nutri.* 126: 476-480, 1996.

27. Sandstrom, B. and A. S. Sandberg. Inhibitory effects of isolated inositol phosphates on zinc absorption in humans. *J. Trace Elem. Electrolytes Health Dis.*

6: 99-103, 1992.

28. Fox, S. I. Enzymes and Energy. *Human Physiology.* Wm. C. Brown Publishers, Dubuque, Iowa, 1993, 81-82.

29. Ashmead, H.D. Food energy utilization from carbohydrates in animals. Albion Laboratories, Inc. 823827 (5882685). 2001. Utah, Buts et al. *American Journal of Physiology,* vol. 251, 1986 G736-G743. 1-22-1992. Ref Type: Patent

30. Ashmead, H.D., D.J. Graff, and H. H. Ashmead. Intestinal Uptake of Free Metal Ions. *Intestinal Absorption of Metal Ions and Chelates.* Springfield, Thomas. 1985.

31. Moran, J.R. and H. L. Greene. The Gastrointestinal Tract: Regulator of Nutrient Absorption. In Shils, M. E., J. A. Olson, and Mike. Hike, eds. Modern Nutrition in Health and Disease. Baltimore, Williams and Wilkins. 1994.

32. Ashmead, H. H. Tissue transportation of organic trace minerals. *J. Appl. Nutr.* 22:42, 1970

33. Graff, D. J. Absorption of minerals compared with chelates made from various protein sources intorat jejunal slices in vitro. 1970. Salt Lake City. 1970. Ref Type: Conference Proceeding

34. Heaney, R. P., R.R. Recker, and C. M. Weaver. Absorbability of calcium sources: the limited role of solubility. Calcif. Tissue. Int. 46: 300-304, 1990.

35. Pineda, O., H. D. Ashmead, J. M. Perez, and C. P. Lemus. Effectiveness of iron amino acid chelate on the treatment of iron deficiency anemia in adolescents. *J. Appl. Nutr.* 46: 2-13, 1994.

36. Ashmead, H. H., Ashmead, H. D., and Graff, D. J. *Amino acid chelated compositions for delivery to specific biological tissue sites.* Albion International, Inc. 826, 786(4,863,898), 1-65. 9-5-2989. Clearfield, utah. 2-6-1986. Ref. Type: Patent

37. Ashmead, H.H. Tissue transportation of organic trace minerals. *J Appl Nutr.* 22:42, 1970

38. Ashmead H., *J. Appl. Nutr.* 22: 42 (1970)

39. Davis CD and Gregor JL, *Amer J Clin Nutr,* 55: 747 (1992)

40. DiSilverstro RT., et al., *J. Amer. Coll. Nutr.,* 11: 177 (1992)